Preggers

By Chelsea Johnson

ISBN 978-0-692-06047-6 (Paperback edition)
ISBN 978-0-692-06092-6 (EPUB edition)

Library of Congress Control Number: 2018901001

Edited by Kirsten Swenson
Front cover image by Stephanie Hansen Photography
"Preggers" title font, King Basil by Missy Meyer
Book design by Chelsea Johnson

First edition, March 2018

Published by Chelsea Johnson
PO Box 43222
Brooklyn Park, MN 55443

Visit www.PreggersTheBook.com

Disclaimer

I am not a doctor, just a mom who loves pregnancy. The information in this book is not medical advice, and it is presented for entertainment purposes only. This book is not intended to replace or substitute for professional medical advice or care, and should not be used for diagnosing or treating any medical conditions. If you have any questions relating to your health or the health of your baby, please consult a qualified healthcare provider.

Table of Contents

Introduction

Hello, Mama! First of all, thank you, thank you, thank you for taking the time to read my book! Whether you got it for your baby shower or your sister-in-law passed it on or you bought it with your own precious money, thank you. It's because of you that this book came to be!

I have always loved writing, but it took me a long time to figure out what I was passionate about. In high school I got voted to be the next J.K. Rowling (although that had more to do with my unmatched obsession with Harry Potter than my writing skills), but I was probably the least likely of anyone at my high school to write a book about pregnancy. Basically, I thought kids were gross and I had never even changed a diaper until my son was born. My mom likes to remind me that I said multiple times that I never wanted to have kids. And yet, here I am with three kids and a pregnancy book under my belt.

Here is a little history about how this book came to be:

When my oldest child was five months old, I started a mommy blog, which I later renamed *Life With My Littles*. I did it just to share some of the tips I was learning about motherhood with other moms, and I quickly realized that people were actually reading and sharing what I wrote. Suddenly, my posts were all over Pinterest and I realized that I could actually write as my job. And then one day I was driving with my kids and I got a sudden desire to write a book. It seemed crazy at first, but I started taking notes about what I wanted to write about and, before I knew it, I had a book outline and ten pages of notes, which turned into this beautiful pink book!

Obviously, this book is about pregnancy and the long nine months it takes to grow a human being. I am going to share advice, tips, and some of my personal experiences. I wrote this like I would write to my sister or a friend, so think of me that way! I'm like your new best friend who gives you support, but will also text you to say that my hemorrhoids are killing me and I just peed my pants a little bit. Think of this book like a pregnancy version of Mindy Kaling's first book (which, by the way, you should all read because it's hilarious and amazing).

This book is also sort of an alternative to a certain anti-vaccine actress' book, which I did not read because I've heard it contains a lot of unnecessary swearing and vulgarity and that's not my thing. I think you can be funny without swearing. But I will be honest and not hold back about some of the more unfortunate, normal things that accompany pregnancy because this book is about every little thing that you might experience. And yes, some of it is gross (have you ever heard of a mucus plug?).

I should let you know that I think I'm pretty funny. So, if it's obvious that I'm trying to be funny and I'm actually not, just save me from any shame and pretend to laugh. Or just don't tell me. That works, too.

Section One has a few serious parts, so it's not as filled with hilarious anecdotes and laugh-out-loud quotes you'll want to text your pregnant sister, but infertility is something I think everyone should be aware of and I wanted to include it in my book.

Throughout my book, I do say "husband" since that's my situation. I know not every pregnant woman is married, but saying "husband" sounds a lot better than saying "significant other," or the much more awkward "husband/boyfriend/partner/baby daddy/sperm donor."

And even though I am married to a doctor, I am not a doctor. So no, this isn't a medical book. Please don't go to your next OB appointment and say, "Well, Chelsea said…." I would be embarrassed for you.

While you are reading, you might encounter things that you haven't dealt with during your pregnancy. But oh man, just because you didn't experience something in your first pregnancy, doesn't mean you won't experience it during your second. Pregnancy is weird like that; you will think you got away with not having morning sickness during your first pregnancy and then it will hit you like a wall during your second pregnancy. Or, as in my case, you might get an insane case of varicose veins during your second pregnancy and be like, "Oh my gosh, what is happening?" So, don't skip sections, okay?

One more thing before we get started. I know pregnancy is an amazing gift and a blessing. I know that not everyone is able to experience it, and even those who do will not experience the same pregnancy. I am in no way trying to hate on pregnancy or say it's something you shouldn't experience. I just want to help other mamas feel like what they are going through is normal and that they aren't alone. Please keep that in mind while you read each chapter.

I love talking about pregnancy and I have a whole lot to say about it, so I hope you enjoy!

Chelsea

Getting Pregnant

Don't Skip This Section!

You might look at this section and think you don't need to read it because you're already cookin'. WRONG. This is the first section of my book because for a lot of women getting pregnant is not as easy as just going off birth control and doing the baby dance a few times. And even if you got pregnant easily, chances are you know someone who is struggling with infertility, or you may even have a hard time getting pregnant in the future. So this chapter is absolutely for everyone.

Many women grow up dreaming of becoming a mother. But nobody tells you how hard it is to make a baby. Getting pregnant with my first baby was one of the hardest things I have ever done. I'm not ashamed of that, and I want to share my story so that others will know they aren't alone.

I want to help raise awareness about infertility because it's not something that women should ever be embarrassed about. Infertility affects 10 to 15 percent of couples in the United States' and is defined as "not being able to get pregnant despite having frequent, unprotected sex for at least a year."[1] If it hasn't affected you, it might be affecting your sister, your best friend, your co-worker, or your neighbor. Infertility is a lot more common than you might think.

Miscarriages happen more than you might think, as well. Sadly, they happen in between 10 to 25 percent of all clinically recognized pregnancies.[2] In other words, up to 1 in 4 women have experienced a miscarriage. I wish it weren't true, but it happens a lot.

Pregnancy happens in a lot of ways. Planned and on the first try, third try, or fifth try. Planned and after using fertility treatments. Not planned and a surprise. Not planned, but not totally a surprise, etc. You get the idea.

We need to support each other and be sensitive about the questions we ask people. One of the worst things you can ask someone is when they are having kids, or if they're going to have more kids. You have no idea what their situation is, and to someone who is struggling with getting pregnant for the first time or the third, being asked when you are going to have a baby is a painful reminder that it still hasn't happened yet.

Even if you get lucky and don't ever have to feel what it's like to struggle with infertility or lose a baby, I guarantee you'll know someone who struggles with this. And if you know what it's like, you'll know how to help them.

Also, there are a few items spread throughout this section that deal with things to do before you get pregnant, what it's like when you think you might be pregnant, and then all the feelings you'll experience when you pee on that tiny little stick. So please, read on.

Things to Do Before You Get Pregnant

I've read tons of books and articles about how to get pregnant, and tons of things about what to do before getting pregnant in order to have a healthy pregnancy. There are actually a lot of things you might not think of that are important to do before you start trying to get pregnant.

I think it's important to know some of these things so you can start your pregnancy off healthy. Pregnancy is not the time to change bad habits. A lot of these are especially important in the first few weeks of pregnancy, and since a lot of people don't know they are pregnant for the first few weeks, you are going to want to do these things before getting pregnant instead of after you're already pregnant.

1. Start taking a prenatal vitamin. This is actually something my husband is a huge advocate of since he is a doctor. All women of "child-bearing age" should be taking a prenatal vitamin. The most important part of the prenatal vitamin is called folate. Folate is super important in the first weeks of pregnancy because it is key in preventing birth defects of your baby's spinal cord and brain. And since birth defects occur in the first 3–4 weeks of pregnancy (aka, before you know you're pregnant), it's important to be taking a prenatal vitamin BEFORE you get pregnant.[3]

2. Lose bad habits. This could be a lot of different things, but I'm mainly talking about smoking and drinking. You can't do either of those things when you are pregnant (duh), so if you want to be a mom and give your child the best start possible, you need to stop those habits before you start trying to have a baby. Drinking increases the chances of stillbirth and miscarriage, can increase your

chances of having a low birthweight baby,[4] can cause fetal alcohol spectrum disorders (that cause developmental and intellectual disabilities), and can cause birth defects like heart defects, or hearing or vision problems.[5] Fetal alcohol syndrome is the only cause of birth defects that is 100% preventable.[6] Smoking during pregnancy can increase the chances of a lot of health problems such as miscarriage, premature birth, and birth defects.[7] So, stop smoking, and if you drink a lot of alcohol, cut back or, ideally, stop. When you are pregnant, you aren't going to be able to do either of those things and still have a healthy baby.

3. Get in shape. If you need to lose some weight in order to be healthy, now is the time. If you don't exercise at all, now is the time to start (but don't start training for a marathon). You can obviously still be overweight and get pregnant, but it won't be quite as easy. Obese women have a higher risk of miscarriage, preeclampsia, gestational diabetes, and hypertension[8], all of which when added on top of other uncomfortable parts of pregnancy, make pregnancy a really difficult time. And if you aren't taking care of yourself during pregnancy by eating healthy and working out, it's going to be a lot harder for you after your baby is born. So get in shape before you start trying to get pregnant. It will make a huge difference in how comfortable your pregnancy is.

4. Stop taking birth control. I feel like this should be obvious, but most doctors recommend stopping your birth control a few months before you start trying to get pregnant. Most doctors actually say stopping 2 to 3 months before trying is the ideal time to stop. It takes a while for the medicine to get out of your system, and you can use other methods of birth control until it's time to start trying ("Yay, condoms!" said no person ever.).

5. Slow down on the caffeine. Caffeine is not recommended during pregnancy, and avoiding it is your safest option.[9] Sorry, mamas, but if you are a huge coffee drinker, try to limit yourself to one cup a day at first, and then find something else to help give you more energy (like exercise). Caffeine is a stimulant for you, and it can be a stimulant to your baby, as well. I have heard that one cup of coffee a day is fine, but the American Pregnancy Association says no caffeine is a much better option. So, slow down on it, and then cut it out. You will have a healthier pregnancy, and you can find other, safer ways to get an energy boost if you need one (But be warned, pregnancy makes you tired either way!).

6. Check your insurance. Being pregnant and having a baby can be expensive if you don't have good insurance, so check yours and see what kind of things it covers in terms of prenatal care and delivery. You want to know exactly what they're going to cover, and what you're going to have to pay. Having a baby can be expensive, so you want to be prepared. And you should also see if your insurance covers screenings and diagnostic testing (like amniocentesis, blood tests, or chorionic villus sampling) for genetic diseases. That way, when you do get pregnant and your OB asks you if you want the tests, you will know if you are going to be paying for them out-of-pocket or if your insurance will cover them.

7. Check your medications. If you are taking something that is not recommended during pregnancy (as a lot of things aren't) then you might want to start going off of it and switching to something that is safer. Talk to your healthcare provider if you aren't sure because he or she will know. I have insane allergies (I'm basically allergic to nature) and I had to stop taking the medicine I was on and find a safer alternative that I could take during pregnancy.

It's always best to stop taking something that could be harmful before you get pregnant.

8. De-stress. Stress isn't healthy in any situation, pregnancy included. High levels of stress over a long time (even a few months) can increase your chances of having a premature baby or a low-birthweight baby.[10] So figure out what is causing you stress and find ways to eliminate those things (if possible) or relieve that stress in a healthy way. If yoga or pilates are not your thing, maybe reading or writing is a good way for you to unwind and relax at the end of the day. Everyone is different, so find something you can do every day to eliminate the bad stress in your life. You will relax and be happier, and baby will be healthier when the time comes!

9. Go to the dentist. Hormonal changes during pregnancy can increase your risk of getting gum disease, so before you decide to get pregnant, go get a checkup! It's also recommended that routine dental treatment is only given in the second trimester as a precautionary measure,[11] so if you haven't gotten your teeth cleaned in a while, getting it done before you are pregnant is your best bet.

10. Clean up your diet. If you eat a ton of fast food, lots of junk food, and not a lot of fruits and veggies, you might want to think about cleaning up your diet before you get pregnant. Your baby gets his nutrients from what you eat, so you want to give him the best, right? And since it's obviously hard to just immediately change your diet when you find out you are pregnant, it's best to work on it before you get pregnant. You should eat a variety of foods to get all the nutrients you need,[12] so eating fast food all the time isn't going to cut it. One way to make it easy is to pretend like you are pregnant and make better choices for the baby that is (soon going to be) in your belly.

Getting healthy and taking care of yourself before you get pregnant is almost as important as it is during pregnancy. And it's a lot easier to start making these changes before you are pregnant so you can give your baby the best start (because otherwise you might gain 50 pounds and that sucks, trust me). You won't even know you are pregnant for the first few weeks, and since that's one of the most important times developmentally for your baby, you want to make them the best few weeks, right? Yes, you do. So do these things and you'll be all set and ready to make a baby!

What It Feels Like When You Can't Get Pregnant

"When are *you* going to have a baby?" she asked me hopefully. There was no malice in her voice, her eyes were full of excitement, and she was clearly just asking a question to make conversation.

"Oh, I don't know. We'll see," I shrugged, giving a polite smile and quickly changing the subject.

To someone who has never struggled with infertility, a simple question about someone's future children seems so innocent. But to someone who has been trying to get pregnant for months, it is a heartbreaking reminder of your ongoing battle to make a baby.

After the first few months of trying, you start to wonder if something is wrong. You record your basal body temperature every morning to see when you are ovulating and use ovulation predictor tests every month so you have sex at the right times. When that doesn't help, you might seek fertility counseling and have lots of hormone tests done. Your husband will get tested, too, to make sure he isn't part of the problem. But when everything comes up fine, your doctors say sorry and tell you to come back after you've been trying for a year.

Each month you have very calculated sex during ovulation, and then wait two agonizingly long weeks to see if it worked. You want to get pregnant so bad that you convince yourself that you're nauseous or extra tired or that your boobs are sore. That makes it even worse when the pregnancy tests are all negative and then the month ends in your period.

When you can't get pregnant, it feels like all of your friends are getting pregnant and leaving you behind. You watch their bellies grow and their babies be born, and as much as you want to be happy for them, you feel like crying every time they post a new picture of their perfect baby.

After a year, when you are clinically "infertile," doctors will start talking about other options. Ovulation medication, fertility treatments, hormone injections, and on and on. You start seriously considering expensive fertility treatments and wonder how much you can afford to spend to make a baby.

The question, "When are you going to have a baby?" is just a reminder that your body isn't working the way you want it to. It is a reminder of the roller coaster of emotions you ride every single month. It is a reminder of all the days and nights you spend crying because it still isn't happening. It is a reminder that what you want the most is to experience pregnancy and hold your own newborn baby in your arms. It is a reminder that you have no idea when you are going to be able to have a baby.

But that's not something you mention in casual conversation. When someone asks, "When are you going to have a baby?" you don't unload the stress you've been feeling for months, or even years, about the pain you've felt while trying to get pregnant. You can't tell them about the battle you've been having with your own body, because if you try, you're just going to break down. So you act casual and brush it off with an "Oh, I don't know. We'll see," and then quickly change the conversation.

It took my husband and me 15 months to get pregnant the first time, plus a round of ovulation medication, and an IUI (intrauterine insemination). But for some women, it takes longer. Some women struggle for years.

So, don't ever ask someone when they are going to have kids. Don't judge someone for having a job instead of having kids, or traveling instead of having kids. You might think they have their priorities mixed up, but they might be going through the biggest struggle of their lives, or maybe they just aren't ready for kids. Either way, it's not your decision, and it's not your place to question them.

And if you're the one who keeps getting negative pregnancy tests, you are not alone. If you are the one who feels like she is bipolar because of the ups and downs of trying to get pregnant, you are not alone. If you are the one who can't look at social media because every time you see another friend's pregnancy announcement you cry, you are not alone.

You are not alone. And you should never feel like you are.

My Personal Experience with Infertility

When my husband and I got married, I had been on birth control for a few months. I took the pill for about a year before I stopped taking it and we started trying to get pregnant. I knew I wanted to be a mother, so I was trying to get my husband on board only a few months after we got married. Having a baby is a big decision, and the timing is different for everyone. We prayed a lot and talked about it and really took it seriously. When we finally both felt that we were ready to start our family, we started trying to get pregnant. It took us 15 months of trying, plus recording basal body temperatures, using ovulation predictors, fertility counseling, several doctor visits, tests for both my husband and me, a round of ovulation medication, and an IUI before I finally got pregnant.

Trying to get pregnant for us was physically demanding because of all the things we had to do, but it was mostly hard because it was so emotionally draining. I felt like each month I was on a roller coaster. I got so excited when I was ovulating and felt so hopeful that maybe this time it would happen. Then it would all come crashing down with a negative test and my period each month. Fifteen months we went through that. I don't even know how many times I peed on a pregnancy test. We could have just waited to find out if I missed my period each month before testing, but anyone who has ever tried to get pregnant knows how eager you are to find out if you are going to be parents. I spent a lot of days and nights crying because it still wasn't happening.

For the first two years we were married we lived in Provo, Utah, where we were both attending Brigham Young University. So, for almost the entire time we were trying

10

to get pregnant, we attended church with other married students where every other girl was getting pregnant and having a baby. I am not saying that it is bad that a lot of young couples want to start families quickly. We did, too. It just makes it ten times harder when it seems like all of your friends are getting pregnant and you keep seeing negative pregnancy tests. And since infertility isn't something you casually mention in a conversation, you just suffer through it together with your husband while everyone else is being blessed with the one thing you want most in the world.

When we graduated from BYU we moved to Colorado for a few months before my husband started medical school. It had been over a year, and we decided to go visit a fertility specialist. She set us up with an ovulation medication and we decided to combine that with an IUI treatment. An IUI is basically where your husband makes a "deposit" in a little cup, then the lab techs separate all the healthy swimmers from the seminal fluid, and then the doctor gets a big turkey baster and squeezes them all up inside of your uterus so they have a better chance of making it to an egg. I know it sounds weird but it's not that strange. Anyway, after it was done, we went home and waited two weeks.

When we finally took a pregnancy test, there was a tiny, faint second line and we knew that it had finally worked.

Fifteen months felt like a long time to me, and I know that for some women it takes even longer, or even not at all. Everyone will have trials in their life that will have to be dealt with, and for me at that point, making a baby was the hardest thing I had done. But our little boy was born safe and healthy four days after his due date and it was well worth the wait.

Am I Pregnant? Phantom Pregnancy Symptoms

When you think you might be pregnant, your mind plays all kinds of tricks on you. You think you are extra tired, or that your boobs feel a little sore. Maybe you feel kind of nauseous, but you were just in the car so you don't know if it's because you might be pregnant or because your mom drives like a crazy person (true life). Or maybe you just threw up that delicious bag of movie theater popcorn on the backseat of your mom's car where you, your husband, and your little sister were riding (again, true life) and you're obsessively wondering if it's because you're pregnant.

Even before we were trying to get pregnant and I wanted to get pregnant, I would sometimes convince myself that I was experiencing early pregnancy symptoms. If I was even close to the end of my cycle, I would start thinking that I was feeling sick or tired or peeing a lot. It was like an obsession I had that I couldn't get rid of.

I specifically remember one time I was at the restaurant where I worked as a server telling my co-worker that I thought I was pregnant because I had been super sick recently. First of all, I was on birth control. Second of all, I had just barely had my period. Third of all, I had no idea what I was talking about, but I wanted to be pregnant so bad that I convinced myself I was. It's madness, guys.

It's especially bad if you've been trying to get pregnant for a while and haven't gotten a positive pregnancy test yet. You might buy a pregnancy test just to be sure, and then when it comes back as negative, you just say, "It's just too early to tell." But, of course, it's because you really aren't pregnant, and you just can't admit that to yourself.

Phantom pregnancy symptoms are real, and they are enough to make anyone crazy. But one day they'll be real pregnancy symptoms and you'll pee on that little stick and you'll feel very justified that you had to take two naps that day.

Reading the Pregnancy Test

I am not one of those girls who doesn't tell their husband that they think they are pregnant and then goes and secretly buys a test and shares the good news in a cute way. I think it's a fun idea, but I just can't keep my "Am I pregnant?" thoughts to myself. My husband always knows, sometimes even before I do.

And my husband also is not one of those guys who jumps for joy when I suddenly tell him I am pregnant without any warning. He needs some time to mentally prepare. Which is understandable, because it can definitely be a big change if you aren't already in the baby mode.

In our house, we have agreed that we buy the test together (and usually a giant drink that I chug on the way home), then I pee on the stick and leave it on the bathroom counter, and we sit in the bedroom for the appropriate three minutes before he goes in and reads the test first. He thinks it's "good luck" that he reads it first, and I don't disagree because I think it's cute that he thinks that ("awwww!").

I did break that rule once (you'll read more about that in a minute) and it didn't go super well.

However you decide to do it, make sure you're not going to embarrass, terrify, or shock your husband, especially if he's in public, and especially if he's at work. That's not how you want to remember the moment you both found out you were going to be parents.

The Day We Found Out We Were Pregnant (Part One)

The first time I got pregnant we had been trying for 15 months. I had peed on a lot of pregnancy tests and seen a lot of lonely lines. The novelty and excitement of peeing on a stick disappeared after the first few months and it had just become a pointless routine for me.

But we had done something different this time (i.e., ovulation medicine and an IUI) so I was a little more hopeful than I had been for the last few months. And I know my husband was, too. We were living with my parents after graduating from BYU and everyone knew we had been trying to get pregnant.

We bought a pregnancy test and waited until the day that our doctor told us to test. I went into our private carpeted bathroom while my husband waited in the bedroom. I opened the test and went through the same boring routine of peeing on a stick. Which, by the way, is super gross, but slightly better than peeing in a cup and then using a dropper to drop a few drops of pee onto a test. Okay, it's a lot better. But I digress.

I peed on the stick and then set it on the bathroom counter while I washed my hands, trying to avoid looking at the test. I nervously went into the bedroom and sat on the bed next to my husband. We waited in silence and kept checking the clock until three minutes had passed.

When my husband slowly got up to go look at the test, I prepared myself to hear that it hadn't worked and that we

14

were going to have to try again. Months of disappointment had taught me not to get too excited.

It was silent for a second and then he turned around with tears in his eyes and told me it was positive. I immediately started crying and said, "Really?" as I got up to look, too. There, on that little stick, was one dark line and one tiny, little, faint pink line: a positive test, finally.

My husband asked me if it was still positive even though it was super faint, and after I told him yes, we just stood there hugging and crying for a while.

We called the doctor and told the nurse the news and were told to come in for a blood test that day just to confirm it. After the test we went to lunch and Babies 'R' Us and bought a pacifier, our first baby item.

The next day, while we were helping pack up my dad's office so he could move to another location, I missed a call from the doctor. I went into the hall and listened to the voicemail where the nurse confirmed that my HCG levels were rising and we were indeed going to be parents. As soon as I shared the news with my husband, we told my family and we all just cried.

I still have the voicemail on my phone. I don't think I'll ever delete it. That was one of the happiest memories I have.

It's Okay to Have All the Feels (Part Two)

With our second baby, we hadn't really been trying but we also weren't not trying (so no condoms, but I also wasn't paying attention to my cycle). Our son was ten months old, and I had just stopped nursing him two months earlier. We also weren't really expecting anything to happen since it had taken us so long to get pregnant the first time.

We got home from Christmas vacation and I had been experiencing those wonderful phantom (or so I thought) pregnancy symptoms we talked about. We heard on the news that there was supposed to be a bad snowstorm the next day that could snow us in for a while, so I suggested that we go to the store and get a pregnancy test just in case we couldn't get out the next few days. My husband agreed (even though I was only like two days away from my period so we totally could've waited) and we headed to the store for a test.

When we got home, we put our son down for bed and I took the test and left it on the counter like we did the first time. I wasn't expecting anything, but I sort of took my time washing my hands and when I looked down, there it was: two dark lines, a positive pregnancy test.

I walked out of the bathroom and told my husband, who was visibly shocked. I was excited, but also didn't feel ready. It was a lot different than when we found out the first time, and I had all the feels.

I was worried about having two so close together (18 months, in case you're doing the math). I was scared how I would handle it with my husband busy in medical school. I felt unprepared and worried that we wouldn't be able to handle it financially. I felt shocked that it had happened so quickly and without any help. I was grateful that it had happened so quickly and without any help. I was excited to see my son as a big brother. I was worried we wouldn't have room in our tiny, two bedroom apartment. Like I said, I felt all the feels.

I'm sure my husband did too, because we sat down on the couch and watched a movie and barely said anything for an hour and a half. But at least there weren't any tears.

It's Okay to Be Scared (Part Three)

The third time I found out I was pregnant was a completely different story. Neither of us was ready for another baby. We had discussed it and decided to wait a while. We didn't want another baby as close as our first two were, and with my husband starting his medical residency, we felt like that first year would be a bad time to have a baby. I was a little sad, but I was at peace with the decision and knew I could be patient until we were ready.

A week earlier, I had published a blog post about getting negative pregnancy tests and what to do when that happens. I had bought a few pregnancy tests so I could get a picture of a negative one for the post picture. Thinking it was impossible I could be pregnant, I opted to run the test under water to get the negative result and then took the picture. I stuffed the other two tests in the back of my bathroom cabinet and didn't think twice about it.

Two days after we got home from my husband's medical school graduation, I still hadn't gotten my period. In fact, I was three days late. I thought it was weird because I usually had a pretty regular 27 or 28 day cycle. But when I woke up early I decided to take a test, even though we had used birth control during the time I was supposed to be ovulating.

Preggers

As soon as I peed on that little stick, there was a little plus in the result window. Hands shaking, I just sat there, stunned. I was completely caught off guard, terrified to tell my husband, and very unsure of what to do. We hadn't planned for this, we weren't ready, and while I love pregnancy and babies and motherhood, I wasn't ready to go through it for a third time just yet.

I dropped the test on the bathroom floor and crept into our bedroom where my husband was still sleeping. I gently moved him and told him he needed to come into the bathroom because I needed to show him something. I'm sure a positive pregnancy test was the last thing he expected. It was the last thing I had expected, too.

I picked the test up with my hands still shaking and showed it to him. Now both in shock, we just stood there confused and worried, the soon-to-be-outnumbered parents of three. I felt guilty that it had happened without us even trying because my sister had been trying for over a year with no success. How could I be pregnant when she wasn't? It didn't seem fair.

The whole day went by in a blur of trying to wrap our heads around what was coming and how our lives were suddenly so different from the day before. It definitely took a while for the excitement to kick in the third time, but that's okay.

Sometimes getting pregnant is unexpected. Sometimes you feel joy and happiness but also fear and worry all at the same time. That's totally okay, and perfectly normal. Becoming parents is a big deal, and luckily, you have nine months to adjust and prepare for the change.

Don't feel guilty if your first instinct isn't to jump up and down. That's not everyone's first reaction. But you should know that there isn't anything that has matched the joy I have felt becoming a mom every single time. Those little stinkers are hard and smelly and wet, but they are so much fun. And whether you're ready or not, they come! So cheers (with sparkling cider, of course) to the next eight months! It's going to go by way too fast.

1. "Infertility." *Mayo Clinic.* 02 July 2014, www.mayoclinic.org/diseases-conditions/infertility/basics/definition/con-20034770.
2. "Miscarriage: Signs, Symptoms, Treatment and Prevention." *American Pregnancy Association.* Aug. 2015, americanpregnancy.org/pregnancy-complications/miscarriage/.
3. "Folic Acid and Pregnancy." *WebMD.* www.webmd.com/baby/folic-acid-and-pregnancy.
4. "Drinking Alcohol during Pregnancy." *BabyCenter.* www.babycenter.com/0_drinking-alcohol-during-pregnancy_3542.bc.
5. "Alcohol during pregnancy." *March of Dimes*, Apr. 2016, www.marchofdimes.org/pregnancy/alcohol-during-pregnancy.aspx.
6. "Fetal Alcohol Syndrome." *American Pregnancy Association*, 1 June 2017, americanpregnancy.org/pregnancy-complications/fetal-alcohol-syndrome/.
7. "Smoking during Pregnancy." *WebMD.* www.webmd.com/baby/smoking-during-pregnancy.
8. Krieger, Ellie, RD. "Plus-Size and Pregnant: The Health Risks." *Parents.*

www.parents.com/pregnancy/my-body/fitness/plus-size-and-pregnant/.

9. "Caffeine Intake During Pregnancy." *American Pregnancy Association.* July 2015, americanpregnancy.org/pregnancy-health/caffeine-during-pregnancy/.

10. "Stress and Pregnancy." *March of Dimes.* Jan. 2012, www.marchofdimes.org/pregnancy/stress-and-pregnancy.aspx.

11. "Dental Care and Pregnancy." *WebMD*, 16 Mar. 2016, www.webmd.com/oral-health/dental-care-pregnancy.

12. "Eating Right When Pregnant." *WebMD*, 26 June 2016, www.webmd.com/baby/guide/eating-right-when-pregnant.

The First Trimester

Congratulations!

Yay! You're going to have a baby! A half-you, half-your husband little person is cooking in your womb! Weird, right? Yes, it kind of is. Technically you've been pregnant for four weeks already when you find out you are pregnant (how confusing is that?), so you've got eight months ahead of you to get ready for your little bundle of joy.

Being pregnant is something to be celebrated because it's the one time in your life that you pretty much have an excuse for everything (we'll talk about that later) and when everybody is super nice to you. Yes, it has rough patches and your body will be unrecognizable by the end, but it's amazing.

But now that you know you're pregnant, what are you supposed to do? What should you expect during the first trimester, and what kinds of decisions do you have to make right now?

In this section all about the first trimester, aka the trimester that you feel pregnant but don't show it, I'm going to answer all your questions: what is normal, what symptoms you might experience, what you should look for in a healthcare provider, and how to decide when to tell people you're pregnant. Most decisions like that are very personal, so weigh all your options and make the best decision for you. It might be different than what your best friend or your sister decides, and that's okay. Your pregnancy is going to be different from theirs so of course your decisions might be different, too.

Are you ready? Here we go!

Things to Do When You Find Out You Are Pregnant

The second you find out you are pregnant, a lot of things can run through your mind.

"We are going to be parents!"
"Oh my gosh, we are going to be parents!"
"We are going to have a CHILD."
"I am going to get so huge."
"It's going to cost so much money."
"I've never changed a diaper before."
"But we are going to be parents!"
"What in the world do we do now?"

During my first pregnancy, I was so full of excitement that I didn't think about some of these things. But after my second pregnancy, I realized that there are several things that you will want to do as soon as you find out you are pregnant, and then throughout pregnancy. I'm including them in the first trimester section so that you can be prepared.

1. Decide when to tell people. This is a very personal decision and I know a lot of people disagree with what I'm about to say, and that's fine, but it's a good idea not to

tell the whole world until after the first trimester is over. I know it can be incredibly hard not to tell your friends as soon as you find out you are pregnant. One thing I worry a lot about is having to go back and tell people that something has happened and I've had a miscarriage. The baby is most vulnerable during the first 12 weeks you are pregnant, and after the first trimester, the chance of a miscarriage drops dramatically (down to 10% of all known pregnancies[1]).

Excuse me while I rant for a minute, but I wrote about this on my blog and got a lot of negative responses from people saying that I was shaming people who have miscarriages and telling them not to share their grief and the loss of their baby. That is NOT TRUE. Let me explain myself.

Miscarriages are awful and incredibly sad. I know they happen and some people handle them better emotionally than others. I am not discouraging talking about miscarriages. I just believe people should at least think about waiting to share their news until the second trimester.

With all of my pregnancies, we told our families that we were pregnant before the second trimester. We told our families we were pregnant the first time right after we had it confirmed by the doctor, our families the second time when I was 8 weeks pregnant, and the third time when I was 12 weeks pregnant. But we didn't announce any of my pregnancies to everyone else until I was in the second trimester (13 weeks).

Like I said, the chance of having a miscarriage drops from up to 25% to 10% when you hit the second trimester. It's still possible to have a miscarriage, but because the chances are lower, I personally think 13 weeks is a better time to announce your pregnancy to the world.

I'm guessing you probably have friends and followers on social media that you maybe met once or twice, but probably won't ever see again. You're probably friends with people from high school that you haven't spoken to since graduation. That's a pretty common thing. The problem that I foresee with announcing your pregnancy before the second trimester is that if something does happen, you then have to go back and tell people you rarely talk to that you lost the baby, over and over again.

I would so much rather just tell my family and close friends because that's where my support system lies. Not in my Facebook friends I never talk to, and not in my Instagram followers I've never met. My family and close friends are the ones I want by my side in the event of a miscarriage, and I don't want random people telling me they are so sorry for me through an online message or comment.

I think it's completely fine if you want to mourn the loss of your baby publicly. It's not shameful to have a miscarriage; they are very common. I am not trying to say that we need to hide miscarriages, but if it was me, I would hate to have to tell people over and over again that I lost the baby and reopen that wound again every time. I would rather talk about it when I was ready, on my own terms.

You may be ready to talk about your miscarriage right away, but you also may not be ready for a month, a year, or even longer. When you wait until your second trimester to announce your pregnancy, you're giving yourself the power to choose when or if you want to share that painful experience, should anything happen.

Yes, you can lose your baby at any time. You might be in that horrible 10% of women who lose their baby after the first trimester. And that sucks.

The decision of when to tell people you are pregnant is personal, and it is different for everyone. But this is my book and I am going to share my advice and my opinions, even if people disagree. Because I really do think that when you find out you are pregnant, it's one of the first things you need to decide. Personally, I would wait until after the first trimester, but everyone can make her own decision.

2. Document your pregnancy. With all three of my babies I took pictures every few weeks. It was so fun to watch my belly grow with each photo. Your body goes through some incredible changes during pregnancy, and I highly recommend taking photos to document it. With my first baby, I took pictures holding a sign each week. With my second baby I uploaded the pictures to my computer and typed how far along I was on each one. With my third baby, I had a countdown shirt and I marked off each week with a red X. I have also seen pictures where people hold fruit representing the size their baby is that week, ones with a chalkboard where you write the changes you've gone through each week, silhouette photos, and photos just of your growing belly. However you want to do it, decide now so you can get started!

3. Take a before picture. With my first pregnancy, I took a "one month" picture as soon as we found out we were having a baby. With my second, I took a "five week" picture. It was fun to see how much different I looked, and

then to compare the before picture with a picture from right before my son was born and then after I had lost the weight. "That will make you feel bad," you may say. No. Trust me. It will be fun to compare, and in my case, it actually helped motivate me to lose the weight once baby was born. And while not everyone may think this is funny, it was crazy to see where I had gained 50 pounds with my son (we'll talk about this later). Unfortunately, my butt was like twice as big and my face was definitely more full. Pregnancy is a strange thing. But then again, when you gain 50 pounds it's not all going to be in your belly!

4. Use lotion early and everywhere. During my first pregnancy, my skin decided that it was going to have stretch marks all over (and I mean all over). My chest, my thighs, my butt, and yes, my tummy. It was probably worse than it could've been since I gained so much weight so fast, but it happened. So, as soon as I started seeing those little lines, I started slathering on stretch mark lotion , and while I still had the stretch marks, I think it definitely helped minimize the long-term effects. So, my advice would be to use lotion early and everywhere because you don't know where you are going to get those stretch marks, especially if it's your first pregnancy. You will go through a lot of it and it's not the cheapest stuff, but it really is worth it!

5. Find a workout plan and stick to it. Not only is it important to workout when you aren't pregnant, it's important to stay healthy and workout while you're pregnant! Your body is going through a lot of changes and you want to keep it healthy. Remember that pregnancy is not the time to start an intense exercise regimen or to lose weight. When I was pregnant the first time I used the stretches and exercises in the *What to Expect When You're Expecting* book and I did them every day. They helped me

stay flexible and I think especially the ones that strengthen your pelvic floor helped me have a really fast delivery. But it was just stretching and not any cardio or strength training, so with my second pregnancy I did a combination of the *FitPlan Pregnancy Journal* and online pregnancy workout videos. I felt so much better doing that than just my little stretches. I recommend a combination of cardio, strength training, and stretching, which will help you stay healthy (as long as you aren't eating too much). If you're already working out regularly (which, bravo if you are), make sure you talk to your healthcare provider to see what is safe to do during pregnancy and if you need to modify any of your exercises. Most things are going to be okay, but every pregnancy is different so it's good to double-check. I also really think that if you are used to working out every day, once you have had the baby it's easier to lose the weight.

6. Research baby products, especially the big things like strollers, car seats, and cribs. One of my favorite places to look (not necessarily buy) is Amazon.com. They have such a wide selection of items, and they have tons of great, helpful reviews for each product. You should also ask any young moms who have recently bought things and see what they like and don't like. And once you do have a few in mind that you feel good about, try and see them in person at the store. I mean really, you have nine months to find these things and you obviously want the best for your child. And the second time around you will already have a lot of the bigger things and won't have to look again. So do your research and you won't have to worry if you're getting what's best for your baby.

7. Make a list of what to do before your baby is born. This was super helpful to me because it helped me feel more prepared before my son was born, and then I knew exactly

what I needed to do after he was born. My list of things to do before your baby is born is coming later in the book, so don't worry about that. Trust me, a lot of good info there. And you don't have to use all of it, but at least add some of the suggestions to your list!

8. Write things down throughout your pregnancy. This can include questions for your doctor, feelings you are having about being a parent, or stories about the firsts (when you first found out, first felt baby, first heard the heartbeat, etc.). These are special things and there's usually a place in the baby book for important dates and how you felt when you found out, so you will want to make sure you remember! And since pregnancy is notorious for making you forgetful, writing down things will help you solve that problem (especially questions for your doctor). Pregnancy is weird and you can easily question the things that are happening with your body. And since you probably don't want to call the doctor every day, write those questions down and bring them to your next appointment. It's super handy to have them right there in front of you when the doctor asks, "Do you have any questions for me?" That way you don't have to be like "Uh, no?" and then remember that you actually had questions as soon as you get home.

9. Start taking a prenatal vitamin. You may already be taking one if you were trying to get pregnant, but if you weren't, start now. They are jam-packed with lots of good things your baby needs to get a head start on life. Folic acid, iron, and calcium are especially important. Prenatal vitamins are not only important for your baby, but they are important for you since your baby is zapping up all those vitamins that you would normally get. You need extra, and that is where a prenatal vitamin comes in. As soon as you find out you are pregnant, get some! And you can

even buy giant bottles that will last all of pregnancy, so that is fantastic. And if taking a pill isn't your thing, now they have gummy vitamins that are delicious and a lot easier to take. So you really have no excuse to get your baby those extra good vitamins and minerals they need while growing!

10. Check your medications to see if you can still take them. I had some allergy medications that I was taking before I got pregnant with my son and after my first appointment, my doctor recommended not taking them anymore. Some things like ibuprofen shouldn't be taken during pregnancy either, so you may want to consider switching to acetaminophen for any headaches or muscle cramps that get severe. There are other things that you shouldn't take during pregnancy, too, so check with your healthcare provider in your first prenatal visit to find out what you need to be careful of. Your healthcare provider will help you balance the risk of harm to your baby with the need you have for the medicine. Make sure you ask because it's much better to be safe than sorry!

11. Download an app to follow along. I personally love the ones where each week they tell you how big your baby is in terms of fruit. My two favorites have been the "What To Expect Pregnancy" app and the "Baby Bump Pregnancy Pro" app. It's fun having access to daily tips, weekly updates, and discussion boards for people who are having babies in the same month as you. And it's exciting to have it right there on your phone every week so you don't have to go looking it up. Even if you aren't big on reading books, at least you get some tips this way!

12. Read as much as you can. When I was pregnant with my first son I pretty much read everything I could get my hands on about babies and pregnancy. I read *What to*

Expect When You're Expecting, The Happiest Baby on the Block, and a few other books that were about the same thing. Especially if it's your first baby or you haven't been around babies much, you want to get as much information as you can about how to be healthy and help keep your baby healthy and growing and happy, right? Fortunately for me I love to read, so this wasn't hard, but even if you aren't a big reader (which, if you are reading this book you probably are), it's different when it's about trying to raise a child. Parenting can be scary stuff, especially when you are first starting out and have no idea what you are doing (which, spoiler alert, nobody really knows what they're doing). So, go pick up a book and start learning all you can because it really does help!

A Quick Note About Second Pregnancies

When I got pregnant with my second baby, I thought I was prepared for what was coming. I'd already done it once, and I didn't think it could be that different the second time around. Boy, was I wrong.

Pregnancy is never the same twice, and things were a lot different in my second pregnancy than they were in my first (and even in my third, too!). Yes, your body has gone through it already, but that means you'll start showing sooner, you'll get uncomfortable sooner, and you might get some new surprises that you didn't get to experience the first time around (hello, varicose veins). So get ready because the second time is a whole new ride.

How to Choose Your Prenatal Care Provider

So I was originally going to write "doctor" or "obstetrician," but there are so many different options out there for prenatal care that it felt weird to write that.

First of all, no matter what you choose, I hope you feel supported in your decision. We should support every woman in her decision on who to go to for prenatal care, even if her decision is different from what we would choose.

You can pick an obstetrician, a family doctor, or a midwife. There are pros and cons to all three, and you should really pick what feels best to you.

Obstetricians: I have seen OBs for all three of my pregnancies and, for the most part, I've been happy with them. An OB is a doctor who has gone to medical school (four years of school) and has done a residency (four more years) specific to pregnancy and gynecology. If you are going to see an OB, you can go to either one specific one or a group of OBs who rotate so you see them all. One thing I have noticed about OBs is that you do a lot of waiting at your appointments. I know that's just how doctors' offices work, but it can be a pain. I also sometimes feel like you are just a number and with all the OBs I've seen, my time spent with the doctor has been 5-10 minutes of the 30-45 (or more) minutes of waiting. I personally like that OBs are trained in C-sections and other medical complications that can come up during pregnancy, but it really depends on your pregnancy and what you are looking for in a provider. And again, no matter what you decide, you should feel supported and comfortable with your decision.

Family doctors: Again, these doctors have gone to medical school (so that means four years of school) and have done a three year residency in family medicine training, so they are very well educated. I think some of the pros of seeing a family doctor is that you can see them even after your baby is born, and since family doctors see babies and kids as well as adults, you can have them be your baby's doctor as well. This is really nice if you want to build a relationship with your doctor and get to know them well. But, if you have a complicated, high-risk pregnancy, this may not be the best option for you.

Midwives: The more I learn about midwives, the more I like them. I like how much they focus on you, and I have heard that women feel like they are heard and their opinions are taken into account with a midwife. They take more time with you and if you are looking for a more natural birth experience, this might be a good choice for you. Midwives stay with you through the labor process and your relationship is more personal. There are different levels of midwives, and some of them are even trained in nursing, too. They can't perform C-sections and if you have a complicated pregnancy, they might refer you to an OB, but I definitely think they are a great choice for prenatal care (especially if you have a low risk pregnancy and want to have an unmedicated birth). Just make sure you know where they deliver and what kind of support or backup they have just in case you do need to have a C-section.

It can be a hard choice to decide what type of prenatal care provider you want to see. There are lots of options, all with pros and cons. Do your research, check your insurance to see what is covered, and make the decision that is best for you. And if your best friend makes a different choice for her pregnancy, support her. It's what you would want!

Your First Doctor's Appointment

Oh, the glorious, long, and awkward first doctor's appointment. You should call and schedule this as soon as you find out you are pregnant. It will usually happen when you are around eight to ten weeks pregnant, unless you had a hard time getting pregnant, in which case your doctor may want to see you earlier.

This is the super fun exam where you get a pelvic exam, pap smear (if you're due for one), blood tests, urine tests (which happen at every exam), and lots of questions. They, of course, check your weight and your blood pressure, but they also will feel your stomach to see the placement of your uterus and determine if you are measuring the same as your due date. They'll ask when the first day of your last period was, so make sure you figure that out before coming, and they'll ask about any previous pregnancies and do a medical history. Your doctor might talk about options for genetic testing and, if you're lucky, you'll get an ultrasound to see your baby! I've gotten an ultrasound at my first appointment twice, so it really depends on your pregnancy, provider, and your insurance.

If this is your first pregnancy or you're seeing a different doctor than your previous pregnancies, they may talk to you about what to expect, how to eat right, ways to stay fit, and what to look out for. You'll also probably be scheduling out your next few appointments, so make sure you bring your planner or scheduler or whatever you use so you don't have to reschedule later. The first doctor's appointment is a long one, so be prepared to be there for a while.

And if after your first appointment you find that you really don't like the doctor or provider you chose, it's totally okay to switch to a new one before your next appointment! Don't feel like just because you went to a doctor once means you are obligated to go to them again.

You want someone who is going to listen to your concerns, make you feel supported, and is easy to talk to, and if your doctor isn't living up to that, you are definitely allowed to find a new one, even if you are two months away from your due date!

What to Expect in the Beginning of Pregnancy

If this is your first pregnancy, you might be wondering what kinds of things you should expect in your first trimester. Besides the wonderful knowledge that there is a tiny human life inside of you, it's kind of rough. Here's what to prepare for:

1. Nausea. The severity will vary for every woman (and every pregnancy), but most likely you're going to get at least a little bit. And it's going to suck. While it might not send you to the toilet, it's not fun trying to do normal things when you feel nauseous all the time. Morning sickness is real, and it's not just in the morning (I guess "all-day sickness" didn't sound as catchy).

2. Lots of peeing. Thanks to those wonderful hormones and an increase in blood volume, you're going to have to pee a lot. If you haven't told people you're pregnant, this one might give it away. I hope you weren't planning on sleeping through the night anymore because I guarantee you'll be up multiple times to relieve yourself.

3. So many feelings. Feelings of joy that you're pregnant, feelings of fear that you're going to be a parent, feelings of worry that you won't be able to afford it, feelings of excitement sharing the news, feelings of sadness because the puppy on the commercial lost its bone, and feelings that you absolutely cannot explain, simply because you

are pregnant. Get prepared for the roller coaster ride of your life.

4. Bloating. You might look down one day and think that you are starting to show, but guys, it's just bloating. And when your skinny jeans won't fit today when you wore them fine yesterday, it's likely because you're bloated. SO MUCH FUN. A recurring question of the first trimester is "Am I showing, or am I bloated?" And as much as you hope you're finally starting to show, you're probably just bloated. If you look skinnier in the morning than you do at night, you're just bloated. Sorry.

5. Food aversions. When I was pregnant with my daughter, anything red velvet made me feel so sick. I didn't even want to think about red velvet. And it's weird because red velvet is good. My pregnant self just decided that was one thing I couldn't handle. So be ready to feel sick just thinking about foods you normally like for no reason. And even if you want something one day, the next day it might totally gross you out.

6. Food cravings. One of the most well-known things about pregnancy is the cravings pregnant women get. Sometimes they are for weird things (pickles and ice cream) and sometimes they will make you drop everything you are doing and head to the grocery store for a very specific flavor of chips. But they start in your first trimester and they usually don't stop until after your baby is born!

7. Tender breasts. Be careful bumping up against things because it's going to hurt. Even if your breasts haven't started getting bigger yet, they are definitely going to be sore. So wear a super padded bra and just be careful in tight places.

8. Larger breasts. One of the very first things my mom said to me when we told her I was pregnant the first time was that she could tell my boobs were bigger. It's embarrassing and awkward, but it was also true. This is a pregnancy bonus for my fellow smaller-chested ladies (and their husbands)!

9. Fatigue. Making a baby is tiring, even from day one. You're going to want to sleep more and sit down more. And things that didn't tire you out before you got pregnant are going to leave you feeling exhausted (like going up stairs). It's rough, but at least you have an excuse to sleep in and take naps! And if your husband complains that you've been sleeping for 10 hours a day, just tell him he did this to you and you're making his child.

10. Mood swings. I sort of already mentioned this, but you are definitely going to experience some mood swings. You might be super happy one minute and the next feel incredibly sad. Or you might snap at people when they weren't even trying to be mean. Thank you, hormones, for making me feel like a crazy person (just make sure that if you're feeling depressed or having difficulty adjusting to pregnancy you talk to someone about it).

11. Super smelling. If there's something stinky in the trash in the next room, you'll know. We had to start double bagging all of my son's diapers when I was pregnant with my daughter because the smells really got to me. But, at least the good smells also smell extra strong!

12. Lower back pain. Because your uterus is all stretching out and your muscles down there are preparing for what's coming, you're probably going to be feeling some pain in your lower back. Your ligaments are loosening up and, oh

man, you will feel it. One thing that has always helped me out is to lay on a bag of frozen veggies!

13. Congestion. If you have allergies, you may have some idea of what is coming but, if not, I'm warning you now that you will probably turn into an open-mouth breather when you sleep for a few months. Thanks again, hormones.

There are a lot of other crazy things that happen to your body when you're pregnant, and we'll get to those later, but just be ready to feel like your body is turning on you. At least the payoff is pretty good!

Dear Arby's

Dear Arby's on Vista Drive,

Thank you for your incredible mozzarella sticks. When I was pregnant with my son, I basically ate them every day. I gained 50 pounds during my pregnancy, but each bite of fried, gooey cheese dipped in rich marinara sauce was worth it.

Thank you for your workers' kindness. They probably knew what the next order was going to be as soon as they saw my car. They never commented on the fact that I was there two days ago ordering the exact same thing, and they were always friendly when I pulled up to receive my bag of hot, golden, deliciousness.

Little did they know I was in my first trimester and craved their mozzarella sticks like they were manna from heaven.

Thank you for those little coupons on the bag for discounted mozzarella sticks that I think were put there just for me. They truly were a gift.

Thank you for making the world's best mozzarella sticks, and for plumping me up like a pregnant balloon.

Sincerely,

My pregnant self

Ways to Deal with Morning Sickness

Any woman who has ever dealt with morning sickness knows that it sucks. And since morning sickness isn't restricted to only happening in the morning, it can keep you from functioning normally.

I'm lucky in that I never throw up when I experience morning sickness, but I do feel constantly nauseous, and that can be rough. With my third pregnancy, I struggled with feeling like I was going to throw up all the time and also feeling like I could eat a whole elephant all the time. It was unfortunate, to say the least.

So I did some research and found nine ways to deal with morning sickness that really helped me feel better and get through that first trimester.

1. Eat a small snack before bed and before you get up in the morning. For me, this meant keeping some crackers by my bedside and eating a few before getting into bed at night and out of bed in the morning. At night it helped calm my stomach so I didn't wake up in the middle of the night feeling sick, and in the morning it helped put a little

something in my stomach before I got up and started moving around. An empty stomach is always a bad idea during the first trimester.

2. Drink something fizzy and orange-flavored. My favorite thing was IZZE drinks in the Sparkling Clementine flavor. They were bubbly and the flavor wasn't too strong or sugary, so taking little sips really helped me not feel sick. Kind of like when I was little and my mom would mix orange juice and Sprite when I was home sick from school! Any type of orange soda or sparkling water that is orange flavored can help.

3. Crackers. I think crackers should be the official food of the first trimester. Super plain and basic, but they really, really help. Like I said, I ate some before bed and before getting up, and then I usually had a few throughout the day when I started feeling sick again.

4. Eat small meals during the day. And I don't just mean scaling back on breakfast, lunch, and dinner. I mean having more than three (like four or five) small, healthy meals. I found overeating really made me sick, and if I went too long without eating I also got sick (pregnancy is fun!). So small meals throughout the day really helped.

5. Drink ginger ale. Another helpful drink was ginger ale. I heard that eating crystallized ginger candy can help, too, but I tried that in high school once and that stuff is disgusting so there was no way I was doing that. Ginger ale that is actually made from ginger (like Canada Dry) has the same effect, though. Our fridge always had a few cans of this for my poor, little tummy. Again, small sips really help.

6. Mints. Not sure why this one helped, but it did. Preferably in a fresh, minty flavor and not in a fruity or sweet one.

7. Sour hard candy. When I was pregnant with Little J five years ago (that sounds like forever) I used Preggie Pop Drops as a way to deal with morning sickness. With my latest pregnancy, I just used lemon drops. Basically, any sour hard candy can help. I'm not sure why, but again, it helped.

8. Suck on Gatorade ice cubes. If you're having a hard time keeping anything in your stomach, try Gatorade ice cubes. It's an easy way to get some electrolytes in your system, and it's a little easier to handle than just having a drink. Regular ice cubes are great, but when you make ice cubes with Gatorade you get the electrolytes, too.

9. Don't let yourself get too hungry. This is one of the biggest tips I can give you. I think the best way to deal with morning sickness and keep it at bay is to prevent yourself from getting too hungry. I know it can be hard to eat anything if you're feeling super sick, but having something in your stomach will help. Try plain, bland foods and nothing with a ton of spice or flavor. I ate a ton of plain bagels in the first trimester, and it helped a lot. I also always kept a little snack in my bag so if we were out somewhere and I got sick I could have a quick snack and feel better.

10. Vitamin B6. Taking Vitamin B6 has been shown to help decrease nausea during pregnancy,[2] too. I've never tried it, but I know some people swear by it!

Morning sickness is not fun, but there are ways to deal with it that can help prevent it and keep it from getting too bad. Hopefully, if you're suffering through that first trimester, you can use some of these tips and get through it a little easier. And just remember, you're doing it all for your baby!

How to Hide a Baby Bump

If you take my advice and don't share your pregnancy news until after the first trimester, you are probably going to encounter the problem of trying to hide a baby bump. It might be small, or it might be a little more bumpin', but, either way, hiding it is going to be key to keeping your special news a secret.

Not to brag or anything, but since I have hid my baby bumps with all three of my pregnancies until we decided to share, I know what I'm talking about. Whether it's a little bit of bloating or a legit baby bump, you're going to want to dress so you can hide it. And since you probably won't be wanting (or needing) to buy maternity clothes yet, I have some tips on how to keep that sweet little bump from giving you away.

1. Loose tops. Obviously if you're bumpin' out, you're not going to want to wear tight shirts. Luckily loose-fitting tops are in style, so people probably won't question your wardrobe choices.

2. Sweaters. Open sweaters, button-up sweaters, long fringe-style sweaters, or pullover sweaters. They are perfect for looking cute and hiding any bump you may be growing.

3. Layers. The more layers the better. They'll hide your bump without anyone questioning your motives.

Especially because everyone wears layers in the fall and winter. (Sorry, spring and summer preggos!)

4. Ponchos. Ponchos (like the sweater kind, not the rain kind) are perfect for hiding a baby bump because they aren't fitted at all. Plus, they're pretty much like wearing a blanket, and how can you say no to that!?

5. Loose dresses. Loose dresses are perfect because they hide growing bellies, and you can even wear leggings underneath which is nice if you can't fit into your skinny jeans already.

6. Divert attention elsewhere. Do you have some adorable ankle booties people always compliment? Or maybe a bold statement necklace? Anything to draw the eye away from your midsection will help.

7. Tuck in button-up shirts. If you tuck in your shirts, you'll get a little bit of a poof at the bottom where they hang over the top. A very sneaky way to hide a baby bump.

8. Patterns. Patterns are going to make it hard to see any bump you might have, so pattern it up! Stripes, polka-dots, flowers, or plaid, it will all work.

9. Black. Everyone knows black makes you look skinnier, so wearing black to hide your baby bump is going to work wonderfully.

The more of these tips that you can combine the better. And if you're one of those people who wants to avoid buying maternity clothes as long as possible, then you can use some of these tips and wear your regular clothes through the second trimester, too!

Gaining Weight and Body Image

I know that most women don't gain much weight (or any) in their first trimester, but I wanted to include this here because I think it's something women can struggle with throughout their pregnancies.

The recommended pregnancy weight gain for women who have a normal BMI before pregnancy is 25-35 pounds.[3] Regardless of your history, this sounds like a lot of weight.

For someone who has struggled with body image issues, gaining weight during pregnancy can be hard. I struggled with body image issues beginning in high school and never really felt comfortable in my body until after my first child was born. I always felt like I needed to be thinner, even though there were times when I was so skinny it was unhealthy. So when I found out I was pregnant I was torn between wanting to be skinny and feeling like I now had an excuse to eat everything in sight and not feel guilty about it. Not a good combo.

It's a difficult concept for some women to accept that it's okay to gain weight during pregnancy. If you've never struggled with body image issues (but honestly, what woman hasn't at some point), then it might seem obvious that, duh, it's okay to gain weight during pregnancy. But if you have struggled, then it can be really hard to accept.

I worried a lot about not being able to get my body back and about the stretch marks I was going to get. I worried that people would think I was fat and that I wasn't going to look good after my son was born.

During my third pregnancy, I had a friend who was two weeks ahead of me with her pregnancy and was training for a marathon at the same time. She looked AMAZING and was so tiny and slim, even though I was bumpin' like nobody's business. At first I was like, "What the heck!?" but then I realized that we just need to accept our bodies and that they change differently. Your pregnant body may be completely different than your best friend's or your sister's, and that's totally okay. Healthy pregnancies look different on everyone.

The most important thing you have to remember during pregnancy is that you are doing it for your baby. You are putting your baby's health over everything else. You are going to gain weight and that's okay! Pregnant women are beautiful, and you are no exception, Mama! So hang that ultrasound picture on the fridge and remember that you are gaining weight for your baby. Embrace your changing body! It's doing something amazing!

The Two Big Questions

There are two big questions that are constantly on a pregnant woman's mind during the first trimester.

The first question is "Am I showing?" and the second is "Did I just feel my baby move?"

I'm just going to answer them both now. No, and no.

As far as showing goes, you're probably just bloated. Unless you were super skinny before you got pregnant, you probably aren't going to start showing until after the first trimester. If you fit into your jeans one day and then you don't the next, and then you are back in them again a few days later, you're just bloated. It's crazy annoying. The good news is that you can wear maternity pants as early as you want, and nobody can tell you otherwise. With my first pregnancy I was definitely wearing maternity pants in the first trimester, even though it was more because I was bloated than because I had an actual baby bump. And I know you really want to be showing because it's so exciting and you don't want that little bump of yours to be from just bloating, but it is, and you'll have to wait a few more weeks for your real bump to make its debut.

For the second question, you won't feel the baby move until probably between 13-25 weeks[4] depending on if it's your first pregnancy or not. Usually what you are feeling is just gas and, yes, it's super hard to decide if what you are feeling is gas or if it's your baby moving. It will take you a while to figure it out, but once you do you'll be able to identify what's your baby and what's just gas. And don't think that just because it's your second pregnancy you'll be able to determine which is which sooner because that definitely was not the case with me (in both my second and third pregnancies!). Even with my third pregnancy, I didn't feel baby move until I was 17 weeks along. That gas can be a tricky one to sort out, trust me.

Things Your Pregnant Wife Wants to Hear

Alright ladies, now it's time to hand the book to your husband to read. I've got a special little section just for him, and you're going to want to have him read it.

Pregnancy is one of the best and worst times of a woman's life. One minute she is in absolute awe that there is a baby the size of a pea growing inside of her, and the next minute she's crying uncontrollably because she's sweaty, hungry, and her pants won't button anymore (a very bad combination).

And if you're married to a pregnant woman, I'm going to be honest and tell you it's going to be a bumpy ride. Walking the line of what's okay to say to a pregnant woman is a dangerous, rocky road that winds and curves and has sharp drop-offs around every corner. You're a brave man for journeying along with her.

Lucky for you, there is one thing that will ensure you can safely navigate that terrifying road without hitting any speed bumps or slipping off the edge to your doom; just tell your pregnant wife exactly what she wants to hear!

Not sure what that is? Here are some suggestions for you to tuck away and use when the time comes:

Any time: "You look beautiful. Nobody can rock that baby bump like you can, honey."

At 3 a.m.: "Of course I will run to Pizza Hut and pick you up some cheesy breadsticks. I have to work in three hours anyway, so I can just start my day a little early. Would you like ranch or marinara to dip them?"

On a road trip: "We can definitely stop again. I know it's only been ten minutes since we last stopped, but my legs are feeling tight. You can pee again while I stretch them out."

Preggers

Before leaving the house: "Hey, let me tie your shoes. You're making our child, and it's the least I can do so you don't have to bend over."

When she has gas: "It doesn't bother me. I'd be gassy, too, if I had a baby in my belly. Just let them out, sweetie. I'll go in the other room."

Any time she complains: "That sucks, babe. I'm sorry."

When she is sad about her stretch marks: "They make you even more attractive to me because they remind me of all that you're doing for our family. You should be proud of those lines!"

When she can't fit into her regular clothes anymore: "Now you can wear your yoga pants all day long! And if you need to go buy some maternity tops, go ahead and take my credit card."

When she literally can't get up off the couch: "Grab my hands and I'll pull you up. I almost got stuck the other day, too! Maybe we need a new sofa!"

In the middle of January: "Yeah, it is super hot in here. How about we turn on the air conditioning today?"

In the middle of July: "Can I get you a bucket of ice to put your feet in so you can cool off?"

When she's nesting at four months: "I'm excited, too. Let's start putting together baby's crib!"

Any time: "I could never do what you're doing, babe. You're amazing, and I love you!"

When she sleeps for 12 hours: "Are you sure you don't want to sleep another hour? You need all the rest you can get!"

When her feet and ankles are swollen: "You should sit down and relax. Can I rub your feet? And how about a pedicure while I'm at it?"

When she can't get off the couch to get the remote that's five feet away: "Oh, don't worry about it. I'll grab it for you. Would you like to watch HGTV or Food Network?"

When her back hurts: "Why don't I schedule you a prenatal massage?"

When she can't sleep at night: "Do you want my pillow? It might help you get more comfy, and I don't really need one to sleep."

When in doubt, use lots of flattery, justify how she's feeling, and offer to do something for her. And remember, it only lasts for nine months.

Working Through the First Trimester

If you're a working mom or if this is your first pregnancy and you have a job, you will quickly discover that working through the first trimester is serious business. With my first pregnancy I was substitute teaching so I had to fight off morning sickness while trying to corral a bunch of middle-schoolers, and with my second and third pregnancies I worked from home on my blog and had to fight being tired and having no motivation to do anything. Either way, it's hard to keep going like nothing has changed.

You may find yourself having to tell your boss why you're going to the bathroom so much, or having to use your sick days due to severe morning sickness. You might even have to sneak a few snacks in to help you fight nausea between meals or take a nap in your car during part of your lunch break. If you have a desk job, remember to get up and move around frequently and sit in a chair with good support, or you're going to be in pain by the end of the day. The point is, you can definitely get through it, even if it's hard to adjust to your fun, new hormones and crampy uterine muscles. It can be rough, but there are definitely ways to make it easier!

Should I Take That Second Nap Today?

If I had to describe the first trimester in three words, I would absolutely include exhaustion as one of those three words (along with starving and nauseous, because that's a fun combination). Your little baby grows a lot during the first trimester (from basically nothing to the size of a lime or plum). And as you can guess, it takes a lot of energy for your body to help him grow. Most likely, this will manifest itself as you being dead tired all the time. We're talking falling asleep while doing something else in the middle of the day tired. You could take a two hour nap after lunch and still be ready for bed by 7 p.m., which, yes, will probably result in getting made fun of by your husband but, whatever. You might look in the mirror and see bags under your eyes that you didn't expect until after baby's arrival. In each of my pregnancies, I have slept a good 10+ hours almost every night in the first trimester and still felt like I needed to take a nap (or two!) the next day. So if you're anything like me and you feel like a zombie by 3 p.m. even when you already napped earlier in the day, it's okay. Go ahead and take that second nap, girl.

How to Stay Positive During the First Trimester

Let's be honest here. The first trimester of pregnancy sucks. You're sick, you're tired, and thanks to your hormones, you have all the feelings. It can be really hard to stay positive during the first trimester when most of your days are spent camped out with your hair pulled back next to the toilet.

Your body goes through a lot of changes during the first trimester, and it can be quite a shock if you've never experienced it before (or even if it's your second or third pregnancy!). The nausea, the bloating, the peeing, the low back pain, the large and tender breasts. It's crazy. And not to mention the sudden life change. Whether you were planning on getting pregnant or not, things change and your future is drastically different than it was before.

Despite all these crazy things that start to happen the moment you find out you're pregnant, there is one thing that can help keep you grounded and help you stay positive and remember why you're putting yourself through this: you are having a baby.

Maybe it comes from a background of dealing with infertility, or maybe it comes from having people close to me go through infertility and suffer miscarriages, but being pregnant is such a blessing, and even though it's hard, it's something that some women never get to experience, despite years of trying.

Remembering the why of pregnancy can make the first trimester easier to deal with because you can focus on the goal. Sometimes you have to go through crappy stuff to get to the good stuff, and pregnancy is no exception.

So when you are trying to get a good night's sleep but have to wake up six times to pee, remember that you're doing it for your baby.

When you are sitting on the bathroom floor next to the toilet trying to take deep breaths and keep your food down, remember that you're doing it for your baby.

When you can't button your skinny jeans even though they fit fine yesterday, remember that you are doing it for your baby.

When a Budweiser commercial comes on and has a soldier coming home to his family after a tour of duty and you start sobbing and can't stop for 10 minutes, remember that you are doing it for your baby.

When you can't even look at bananas at the store or stomach the smell of banana bread or have to avoid scrolling through Pinterest because seeing banana recipes makes you gag, remember that you are doing it for your baby.

When you can't lay on your stomach to sleep because your tender, growing breasts are way too sensitive, remember that you are doing it for your baby.

The first trimester is rough and it sucks and you're going to look forward to the day it ends, but you are doing it for your baby. And remembering that can help you stay positive, focused, and get through it with a smile on your face. Because your baby is worth it all. And I promise, the second trimester is way better!

1. "Second Trimester Miscarriage." *BabyMed.com*, 26 Feb. 2015, www.babymed.com/complications/second-trimester-miscarriage.
2. "Morning Sickness Relief: Treatment & Supplements." *American Pregnancy Association*, 10 Aug. 2017, americanpregnancy.org/pregnancy-health/morning-sickness-relief/.
3. "Pregnancy Weight Gain." *American Pregnancy Association*, 12 Dec. 2015, americanpregnancy.org/pregnancy-health/pregnancy-weight-gain/.
4. "First Fetal Movement: Quickening." *American Pregnancy Association*, 2 Sept. 2016, 3. http://americanpregnancy.org/while-pregnant/first-fetal-movement/.

The Second Trimester

The Golden Trimester

Guess what!? You've made it to the second trimester! For most women that means peeing less often, no more morning sickness, and getting your energy back. I like to refer to the second trimester as "the golden trimester" because it's easily my favorite of the three. You aren't throwing up anymore and you aren't uncomfortable to the point where you just want your baby to be born already. You've probably found that you aren't as tired and your baby bump is turning into a baby bump and not just a bloat bump. This is also the trimester that you get to see your baby on an ultrasound (if you haven't already, it depends on your doctor and your medical history) and you may find out if you're having a boy or a girl. You'll quickly find, as so many other women have before you, that the second trimester is the easiest and most fun trimester of the three. Enjoy it while it lasts because before you know it, you'll be waddling around getting ready for your baby to come!

How to Announce Your Pregnancy

We've already talked about deciding when to announce your pregnancy, so now let's talk about how to announce your pregnancy!

One of my favorite parts of being pregnant is announcing the big news to my family and friends. Personally, I have always waited until the second trimester for the big reveal. And these days there are so many cute, unique ways to announce your pregnancy that simply saying "I'm pregnant!" just doesn't cut it (obviously this is based on personal preference and if you are someone who is cool with a simple announcement, no judgment!).

My favorite (and probably the easiest besides just saying that you're pregnant) way to announce your pregnancy to the world is with a cute picture. Just a quick search online (or of my blog!) reveals tons of clever ways to share the news with a photo. You can use just the pregnancy test, your pet, older siblings, a pregnancy book, baby clothes, baby shoes, foods you're craving, a bow around your belly, signs, chalk, Prego pasta sauce, a stethoscope, an ultrasound picture, or even balloons. There really are so many adorable props you can use to take a pregnancy announcement picture. I've also seen cute videos of people announcing their pregnancies, so if you want to put a little more time and effort into announcing, that's another option.

Announcing your pregnancy and sharing the big news is such a fun part of being pregnant, so take advantage of it!

The Awkward "Chubby or Pregnant?" Stage

Now that you are in the second trimester, you are probably actually starting to show instead of just being bloated. It's super exciting and it will make your pregnancy feel even more real. However, there is a stage that lasts for a few weeks where you may feel like strangers are looking at you trying to decide if you are just a little chubby or if you're pregnant. It's not a big deal, but be ready. If it does bother you, wearing loose-fitting tops will help until you feel more comfortable rocking those tight maternity tees. And, don't worry; your baby bump will be super obvious before you know it!

Showing Earlier the Second Time Around

If this is your second (or third or fourth!) pregnancy, you may discover that you start showing sooner than you did with your first baby. This was the case for both my second and third pregnancies. Your once tight ab muscles were loosened the first time around, so the second time around they don't hold your pregnancy in as well.[1] It's totally normal and doesn't mean that your baby is bigger or that you're going to be bigger this time around, either. So don't sweat it!

Myths About Maternity Clothes

When I found out I was pregnant with my first baby, I was so excited that I bought (and started wearing) maternity clothes when I was only 2 months pregnant. You might think that's ridiculous, but after trying to get pregnant for 15 months, I was so ready to embrace every aspect of pregnancy, maternity clothes included.

Even in my third pregnancy, I still loved maternity clothes. I wore them every day and I think they're the bomb. If I could, I would for sure wear maternity pants every day, even when I'm not pregnant. Stretchy waistbands forever!

But if you aren't quite as convinced about the benefits and amazingness (yes, it's a word) of maternity clothes, I'm going to try and change your mind! I know a lot of people like to just wear men's t-shirts and yoga pants until delivery, but I personally wouldn't feel as confident or cute wearing that every day. So, let me tell you six myths about maternity clothes and why they are ALL false! Maternity clothes are a MUST when you're pregnant, so give me a chance to change your mind and show you why you should definitely buy (at least some) maternity clothes when you're pregnant.

1. Maternity clothes are hard to find. FALSE! Maternity clothes are not hard to find at all. A lot of major chain stores have maternity sections so you can try clothes on before you buy them. And then there's the wonderful internet with tons of maternity stores for every style. Some of my favorites are Gap, Old Navy, Target, PinkBlush Maternity, and Zulily. Maternity clothes are everywhere, so don't even try to sneak this little lie past me!

2. Maternity clothes are uncomfortable. FALSE! As soon as you slip into a pair of maternity pants or pull on a maternity shirt, your mind will quickly change on this one. The stretchy waistbands of maternity pants and the extra room in maternity tops are oh-so-comfy. And don't even get me started on maternity dresses. Maternity dresses are amazing, and especially perfect if you live somewhere hot or will be pregnant during the summer. This myth is a big fat lie so stop telling it to yourself!

3. Maternity clothes are expensive. FALSE! I mean, yes, there are some that are on the more expensive end, but that's how all clothes are. There are lots of great places to buy affordable maternity clothes. So no, maternity clothes are not expensive (at least not any more expensive than non-maternity clothes!).

4. You don't need maternity clothes when you're pregnant. FALSE! Oh my goodness, unless you want to wear your husband's extra large shirts and sweatpants during your whole pregnancy, this is not true! You can get away with wearing most of your shirts until maybe the middle of your second trimester, but then you'll start stretching them out and you will probably ruin them and not be able to wear them after pregnancy. So, you definitely need maternity tops. And as far as pants go, you'll probably need to get some maternity pants even before your maternity tops. With all three of my pregnancies, I haven't been able to fit into my regular pants by the beginning of the second trimester. If bloating doesn't make it impossible to button your pants, then the growing baby bump will. You definitely, absolutely need maternity clothes.

5. Maternity clothes are a waste of money. FALSE! Yes, it's true that maternity clothes are only meant to be worn for a few months. But honestly, a lot of them you can wear when you're not pregnant, and you'll probably be wearing them for a few weeks (or maybe months) after your baby is born, too. If you don't have a ton of extra money to spend on maternity clothes, be smart and shop for things that you can wear during pregnancy and when you're not pregnant. And if you are pregnant more than once, then you get to wear them again! I have several tops that I have worn during all three of my pregnancies. Maternity clothes are absolutely not a waste of money.

6. Maternity clothes are ugly. FALSE! This may be the biggest myth on this list because maternity clothes are so cute! There are maternity clothes for every style, and I have a hard time not buying a full wardrobe every time I'm pregnant! Maternity clothes may not have been super cute like 15 or 20 years ago, but now they are adorable and I want them all.

There are a lot of myths about maternity clothes out there, but most of them aren't true. Maternity clothes today are cute, affordable, comfortable, and definitely a must-have when you're pregnant. So stop trying to tell yourself you don't need them because you do!! And I'm sure once you pull on your first maternity outfit you'll be hooked, too!

The Anatomy Scan

Between 16–20 weeks your provider will likely order an ultrasound to perform an anatomy scan. This is the highly anticipated "gender ultrasound" that parents-to-be look forward to. I know a lot of moms who decide to wait and be surprised when their baby is born, but that is just not me. Even when I had one boy and one girl and was pregnant with my third, I had to know what we were having. I'm more of a have-everything-ready-to-go kind of girl than a buy-everything-gender-neutral-and-after-the-baby-is-born-buy-blue-or-pink kind of girl. Either way is fine and it's a personal decision but, like I said, I just have to know.

Make sure your ultrasound tech knows whether or not you want to know your baby's gender before they put the jelly on your belly. I have heard stories about people going in not wanting to find out the gender and then the tech accidentally spills the beans or doesn't warn the parents that she is going to check baby's privates and the parents look at the screen at the wrong time. Oops!

You'll probably notice during the ultrasound that the tech is going to be taking a lot of measurements and moving all around your belly to see every part of your baby. This ultrasound is important because it gives your doctor a chance to see if your baby is healthy and developing the way he should. The tech will look at your baby's head size, leg and arm bone sizes, and heart size. You'll get to see his tiny heart and all four chambers pumping away on the screen.

The anatomy scan is fun, regardless of if you are finding out your baby's gender or not. I have always loved seeing the baby's tiny little bones wiggling around and the tiny hands moving around by the baby's face on the screen. And the full body with the profile shot just melts my heart. It's such a special moment, especially if you haven't had an ultrasound up to this point.

The Gender Reveal

With all three of my pregnancies, I've wanted our baby to be a certain gender. I wanted our first to be a girl because I didn't have any brothers growing up and had no idea what to do with a boy (I quickly figured it out!). Our second baby I wanted to be a girl, too, since our first baby was a boy. And then with our third, I would have been happy either way, but I secretly wanted our baby to be a boy just a tiny bit more. It's hard not to have at least a tiny bit of a preference, even if you don't say it out loud!

After having both boys and a girl, I can tell you that both are amazing. They both have fun things that go with them (trains and trucks or princesses and dolls) and, either way, you will love them with all your heart. The most important thing is that they are yours, and even if you are scared to have one or the other like I was at first, once they are born you will quickly forget all about that and love them for who they are.

If you decide to do a big, fancy gender reveal for friends and family or to share on social media, the options are pretty much endless. Just like announcing your pregnancy, there are tons of ways you can announce your baby's gender. You can throw a party and surprise your guests with a balloon pop or cake reveal, you can take a picture holding a baby boy outfit or a baby girl outfit, you can make a video releasing balloons from a box, or you can even give your kids donuts filled with blue or pink filling like we did for our third baby. A quick search online will reveal tons of ideas, ranging from easy to complicated. I have a few posts on my blog with ideas if you want some inspiration.

No matter what you decide to do, don't let other people pressure you in your decision. It's your choice, and they'll find out eventually whether it's at 20 weeks or when your baby is born!

Things That Happen to Your Body During Pregnancy

Pregnancy is a beast and it seriously takes a toll on your body. You are essentially sacrificing your body for nine months to GROW A HUMAN. And regardless of if this is your first or fourth pregnancy, you might be wondering if the weird things that are happening to you are normal. Don't panic if you start experiencing one of these things because, I promise, it's normal and enough pregnant women have experienced it that it's on this list (aka, you're not a weirdo).

1. Carpal tunnel. This is where you get a pinched nerve and part of your hand or arm goes numb, feels tingly, or is painful. I had it at night when I was pregnant with my first son, and I had to wear a wrist brace when I slept. It went away after he was born. Super weird, super annoying.

2. Acne. Thanks to your wonderful hormones during pregnancy, your face might suddenly look like it did when you were a teenager. The good news is that it will clear up after your baby is born! Just make sure you wash your face every day.

3. Popped belly button. I feel like most people know that towards the end of pregnancy your belly button becomes a super outie. It's super fun (not) when you can see it through all your shirts and people "affectionately" call it your turkey timer.

4. Stretch marks. Not just on your belly, either. Stretch marks can happen on your butt, boobs, and thighs, too. Pretty much anywhere you gain a lot of weight fast. I had them everywhere with my first son (and I mean everywhere).

5. Amazing hair. One great thing that pregnancy does is that your hair gets super shiny and thick and feels fabulous! Because of your hormones, it grows faster and grows wonderfully. You're probably going to want to audition for a few hair commercials over the next few months.

6. Linea nigra. This a vertical, dark line on your abdomen that goes up to your belly button. Not all women get it, but it's a possibility.

7. Waddling. Thanks to the baby positioned down in your abdomen, toward the end of your pregnancy, you start waddling. No more walking normal for you! Husbands think it's super funny and like to make fun of you, but it's definitely not funny. If only they knew.

8. Nausea. The degree of nausea and how long it lasts varies, but in the first trimester (and sometimes into the second), nausea is very common. It sucks, yes, but it usually goes away.

9. Breast changes and tenderness. Sometimes bigger isn't always better because along with the size change, your breasts are going to be tender and even lightly bumping up against something will hurt. Make sure you invest in a good bra because it will make a big difference in your comfort level.

10. Varicose veins. These might pop up in your legs or even in your vaginal area, especially as pregnancy progresses. As the pressure of your baby on your lower body gets more intense, your veins have more pressure on them, and that's when varicose veins happen. I didn't have these when I was pregnant with my first son, but with my daughter, I got them pretty bad in my legs. And then with my second son I got to learn all about vaginal varicosities (more on that to come later). Compression stockings can help, but if you are pregnant during the summer like I was, you might think twice about wearing them.

11. Cankles/swelling. Your hands (goodbye, well-fitting wedding ring), your feet (hello, flip-flops), and those glorious elephant-like cankles. Sexy!

12. Hemorrhoids. Another problem from pressure on your lower body, hemorrhoids can be internal or external.

Hopefully you don't have to deal with these, but if you do, it's normal and they can be treated.

13. Heartburn. The progesterone you are producing relaxes the muscles of your uterus, but it also relaxes the valve between your esophagus and stomach, which leads to acid sneaking it's way out and making you feel like your chest is on fire, even if all you've had is water. Take some antacids and prop yourself up with pillows. It will be over soon!

14. Weight gain. Obviously. I'm not even going to explain this one.

15. Eyesight changes. Those darn hormones are at it again. It's not a big deal and it's usually not super dramatic, so don't worry and don't go buying new glasses. Your vision will go back to normal after your baby is born.

16. Itchy belly. Okay, so I know this isn't a technical term, but with my pregnancies my belly got super itchy as it stretched and my babies got bigger! It's super annoying, and all you can really do is make sure you put lotion all over your belly.

17. Back pain. Especially lower back pain. It's rough and it makes everything uncomfortable (walking, sitting, sleeping, being alive).

18. Gas. It's the worst. And as your abdomen stretches and things down there change, it gets harder to keep it in. And it hurts, too. So you will feel like a balloon sometimes. You better hope your husband is a forgiving and loving man because he's going to get put to the test with this one.

19. Cravings. When I was pregnant with my first son I went through the Arby's drive-thru several times a week because I could not get enough of their mozzarella sticks. And when I was pregnant with my daughter, all I wanted were Pringles. With my second son, I wanted burgers morning, noon, and night. Cravings definitely strike during pregnancy, and it's totally normal!

20. Vaginal discharge. Yup, I said it. It's super gross, and I wish it wasn't so. You'll probably have to have a pantyliner in your undies the whole time you're pregnant, so that's fun (only not).

Learning How to Side-Sleep

Sleeping during pregnancy is basically a joke, and even though the second trimester is better than the other two, it still has a few drawbacks.

I hope you aren't a back-sleeper because when you hit the second trimester, you aren't supposed to sleep on your back anymore. When you sleep on your back, the weight of your uterus rests on your inferior vena cava, the main vein that carries blood back to the heart from your lower body. Putting pressure on this can reduce circulation to your uterus and baby, which prevents oxygen from getting to them[2]. Obviously, not good. And, of course, you can't sleep on your belly because it's getting bigger and that'd be like trying to sleep on a beach ball. So, a side-sleeper you must become.

It definitely takes some time to adjust to side sleeping, and it will be uncomfortable at first if it's not something you're used to. Putting a pillow between your knees and in front of your stomach helps make it more comfortable. And, enjoy it while you can because the further along you get, the worse it's going to be! Just dream of the day when you're finally able to sleep on your belly again! It's magical!

Make Daddy Feel Special, Too!

Even though I mostly focus on all that you can do to make pregnancy special and less uncomfortable for you, I also think it's important to remember that you aren't the only one waiting for your baby! Your husband is eagerly awaiting the birth of your baby, too, and even though he doesn't get to experience pregnancy in the same way you do (no peeing in a cup every month for him!), he's a big part of the process, too! After all, you wouldn't be in this situation without him! So here are some ways you can make him feel special and involve him in your pregnancy.

1. Let him come to appointments with you, or record the heartbeat if he isn't able to make it. My husband has rarely been able to come to appointments (except for ultrasounds), but this is a great way to help him feel involved. Those appointments make the pregnancy feel a little more real, especially when you get to hear baby's heartbeat! If he's not able to make it, record the heartbeat on your phone and play it back for him later. He'll appreciate it!

2. Let him know when the baby is moving so he can feel baby kick. It might be a while before baby is big enough that you can feel him from the outside but, when you can, let your husband know so he can feel baby move, too! I still remember the first time my husband felt our first baby move! It's a moment you'll never forget!

3. Take maternity pictures together. I have seen some beautiful maternity pictures where couples have both been

in the shot, and I love the idea of getting your husband involved in your maternity shoot. We took a few non-professional pictures together with our first baby, and I still love looking back on them! We were so young!

4. Build items (like the crib or swing) together. One of my favorite things to do with my husband when I'm pregnant is get things ready. The first time we put the crib together was so fun! And setting up the pack n' play, the bouncer, and the swing together was fun, too!

5. Register together. If you thought registering for your wedding was fun, just wait until you register for your baby! Diapers, baby monitors, blankets, tiny little outfits, it's a blast. And depending on where you register, you'll probably get a few free goodies, too!

6. Have him rub belly butter on your stretching belly. One of my friends suggested this and I think it's a great idea. Plus, he might get to feel baby kick when he does it!

7. Ask him to massage any sore areas. Another suggestion from my mama friends and I love it! This is especially wonderful towards the end of pregnancy when everything hurts!

8. Gift him a new dad kit. When I was pregnant with our first I made my husband a new dad kit, and he loved it! It was full of little things to help him in his new role as a daddy (like earplugs, energy drinks, and a baby shirt of his favorite football team).

9. Throw a gender reveal party together, or invite husbands to the baby shower. Now that gender reveals are basically all the rage (yeah, I used that phrase like an 80-year-old), a gender reveal party is a great way to celebrate

your baby together! Or you can even invite husbands to your baby shower and let them do their own thing (grill burgers on the deck?) while the ladies hang out and talk about labor and breastfeeding. Plus, that way he can open baby shower gifts with you!

10. Take classes together at the hospital. Another great way to involve your husband in your pregnancy is to go take a baby basics class or childbirth class together at the hospital. We went to one when I was pregnant with our first and it was so helpful to learn all about car seats, bathing, diapering, and swaddling. If you haven't been around babies much, I highly recommend it!

There are many ways to involve your husband in your pregnancy, and I am a big advocate of making him feel like he's a part of your pregnancy, too. Like I said, you didn't get that way on your own, and he's excited to meet your little wee one just like you are!

Ever Had a Charley Horse?

If you've never had a Charley Horse before you are in for a real treat (NOT! Are "not" jokes still a thing?). I've gotten at least one with each of my pregnancies, and they suck. For me, they've happened in the middle of the night in my calves and they've been so painful that I've woken up screaming. I think if you asked my husband he'd probably say Charley Horses are one of his least favorite parts of pregnancy because I scare him so bad and he thinks the worst is happening. Not to freak you out or anything, but it's like a terrible sharp pain in one small place that makes your leg (or whatever body part it's happening in) feel like it's dying. The worst part is that you freeze up and can't move it at all, which is unfortunate because stretching it out is what makes it go away. I've never been able to stretch it out myself, and I've always had to have my husband do it while I'm squirming around in pain. It's the worst. And they're pretty common during pregnancy. Just remember that if you get one, don't lose your crap. Try to remember to stretch it out!

Heartburn (aka Hellfire in Your Chest)

Up until being pregnant, I'd never really experienced heartburn. I thought it was a weird term, and I didn't get why people made such a big deal about it. I was so naïve.

As your pregnancy progresses, those wonderful hormones, combined with your growing uterus squishing your stomach and giving it less space, make your stomach acid splash up into your esophagus. It is especially painful when you eat anything spicy but, honestly, sometimes it doesn't matter what you eat and you'll still feel it: a cookie, a bagel, even a drink of water. They all come back up and burn with a vengeance. At first, just laying down in bed will make it act up. You're not supposed to lay down for an hour after eating, so that makes sense. And don't even think about trying to tie your shoes because bending over makes it 1,000 times worse and you'll be like "WHAT IS HAPPENING!?" Eventually it will hurt no matter what, even if you're sitting completely straight up in bed. Which makes it super fun for sleeping because everyone knows sitting up is the most comfortable position for sleeping. I basically lived with a bottle of chewable antacid on my nightstand the second half of pregnancy.

Have you ever heard the old wives' tale that if you have heartburn during pregnancy your baby is supposedly going to have a ton of hair? I know it sounds like it's probably not true, but there was a legit study done at Johns Hopkins University that showed there is really a correlation between heartburn and the amount of hair your baby has[3]. For me personally, my second and third babies had beautiful heads of dark hair and the heartburn I suffered with those two was rough. I can still feel the fire in my chest thinking about it now.

However, I did do my own little poll of my friends and social media followers, and while a lot of them said that they had horrible heartburn and babies with tons of hair, a lot of them also said that they had bald babies despite horrible heartburn. So, don't get your hopes up that your baby will come out looking like a Troll doll even if you have heartburn! It might not happen!

The Glucose Test

At the end of your second trimester, your doctor is going to have you take a glucose test to make sure you haven't developed gestational diabetes. Basically, you have to drink a super sweet drink in less than five minutes, wait an hour, and then get your blood tested. I've always heard women complain about the drinks but, if we're being honest, I actually enjoy them. I've always chosen the orange flavor and I think it tastes like a super sweet orange Gatorade. If you're worried about it, take the full five minutes to drink it, but it's really not a big deal. I usually down mine in about a minute (CHUG! CHUG! CHUG!).

During my first pregnancy I was a vegetarian, and I'm also allergic to nuts, so if I had failed and had to cut back on the carbs I probably would have died from starvation. I might be exaggerating a little bit, but I was a super picky eater at the time (I have since changed my foolish ways).

If you fail the glucose test, you have to come back and take a three-hour test; if you pass, you're in the clear and don't have to worry (although you should always make smart choices with what you eat during pregnancy, even if you don't have gestational diabetes).

I've had friends who have failed both tests and ended up being diagnosed with gestational diabetes, and while it isn't something to be taken lightly, it can be managed. Make smart choices and listen to your healthcare provider's recommendations so that you and your baby will have a better chance of being healthy.

Feeling Your Baby Move

One thing I hear a lot of women say after their babies are born is that they miss feeling their baby move around inside of them. Yes, of course, it's better to have your baby in your arms and actually be able to hold them, but there's something really special about feeling your baby move when you're pregnant.

At first you'll feel him from the inside, just small "flutters" as they are called. Like I said before, in the beginning it's super hard to know if you're feeling gas bubbles or your baby moving (and you'll have a lot of gas, so that's fun). You'll be all "OMG! I think I felt him! No wait, was that gas? I think that was gas…but there it was again!" It's the worst. But then one day you'll be watching TV or driving in the car and BAM! You'll know without a doubt that it was your baby moving.

As your baby grows, the movements will get a little stronger, and eventually you'll be able to feel him move from outside your belly. It's so fun getting your husband involved and having him feel the baby move, too. Or even better, letting your baby's older siblings feel him move. I'm pretty sure my 3-year-old didn't quite understand what was going on but, regardless, he loved feeling "his baby" move around (and, of course, when your mom visits she'll want to feel baby move, too, because you know, that's just how moms are).

The closer you get to your due date, the more uncomfortable baby's movements will be. He'll kick you in your ribs or stretch and push down into your pelvis and you'll be like "How did I ever enjoy this?" You'll try to massage your belly down to coerce your baby to get out of your ribs and into a more comfortable position. You might even lean over and yell at him to "MOOOOVE!" a few times.

So, enjoy it now in the second trimester because the third trimester is a whole different story!

1. "Pregnant again: What to expect this time around." *BabyCenter*, Apr. 2017, www.babycenter.com/0_pregnant-again-what-to-expect-this-time-around_10305185.bc.
2. "Sleeping Positions During Pregnancy." *What To Expect*, 10 Mar. 2017, www.whattoexpect.com/pregnancy/sleep-solutions/pregnancy-sleep-positions/.
3. Costigan, Kathleen A., et al. "Pregnancy Folklore Revisited: The Case of Heartburn and Hair." *Birth*, vol. 33, no. 4, Dec. 2006, pp. 311–314., doi:10.1111/j.1523-536x.2006.00128.x

The Third Trimester

2/3 Baked

Congratulations, Mama! You've made it 2/3 of the way through your pregnancy! You are so close (even though it might still seem so far away), and before you know it, pregnancy is going to be over! If we're being honest, I've always thought the third trimester was the worst of the three. Your body hurts, you can barely move, you're exhausted, and you just want to meet your baby already. Buckle up because things are about to get REAL.

A Third Trimester Haiku

I have to go pee.

I can't get comfortable.

Pregnancy is fun.

People Don't Ever Know What to Say to a Pregnant Woman

For some reason, people don't always use common sense when speaking to pregnant women. I don't know if people just forget what it's like to be pregnant, forget that you are still a person, or they haven't experienced pregnancy (men, I'm talking to you), but sometimes people do not think through what they say to you when you are pregnant. After three pregnancies, I have gotten my fair share of interesting and inconsiderate comments. I know that people don't do it on purpose, but there are some things you just should not ever say to a pregnant woman.

The first thing people should know when addressing a pregnant woman is that even though she is pregnant and her belly is obviously growing, she does not like any references to her weight gain. I think that's totally justifiable, especially since you're already a little more sensitive when pregnant. Nobody likes to get bigger, even if there is a good (cute baby) reason for it. That being said, here are the worst things to say to a pregnant woman:

1. "You're getting so big!" Yes, dear family members, this one is for you. Yes, every time you see me I am going to be bigger. Babies grow, and since my baby is in my tummy, my tummy is going to grow. Unless you're talking to a five-year-old, this is never an acceptable thing to say.

2. "You look ready to pop!" When you say this to a pregnant woman, it implies that she is almost done with pregnancy. But, oftentimes, she still has several weeks or even months to go. And then when she is almost done with pregnancy, it just reminds her that no, she has not

delivered her baby yet and yes, she is miserably uncomfortable (especially after the due date).

3. "Are you having twins?" Again, this implies that the pregnant woman is huge. And since the likelihood of having twins is very low, it's probably best to just assume there is one baby in there. Also, don't ask "Are you sure?" when the response to this question is "no." You deserve a slap in the face for that one.

4. "You're a lot bigger this time around." This deals with second or more pregnancies (obviously). Saying this makes the pregnant woman think that you think she looked better with her first pregnancy (even if that's not what you mean, pregnant women are often irrational). Yes, she might be bigger with her second or third pregnancy, but don't point that out. It's not very nice.

5. "How long do you think it will take you to lose the weight?" When you are pregnant you do not want to think about having to lose the baby weight. Especially if you gain 50 pounds. It stresses the pregnant woman out and makes her feel like she shouldn't be gaining any more weight because you think she is already a whale. Which you most likely don't, but she will be sensitive and take it that way because, you know, hormones.

6. "You don't look very big. Are you eating enough?" Yup. Now back off while I go throw up again because I have morning sickness from hell.

If you're pregnant (or have been pregnant), chances are you've had to fend off one of these thoughtless comments. Like I said, people just say dumb things to pregnant women because they don't know what it's like to be pregnant, or because they just don't remember how it feels to be pregnant. Or sometimes they are just dumb because there are for sure dumb people out there who just don't think.

Now, let's talk about things that are always okay to say to a pregnant woman. Basically, you want to buoy her up and never mention her size. Here are some suggestions:

1. "You are beautiful/amazing/gorgeous." This is obviously good to say to anyone, but especially good for a pregnant woman. Why? It takes the focus off of how round her belly is getting, and makes her feel good about herself, despite the cankles, weight gain, sweating, and acne breakouts. Anything to make a pregnant woman feel good is a great thing to say, especially when she feels gross and is super emotional.

2. "You are such a cute pregnant woman." I went to a waterpark when I was eight months pregnant and had a lady tell me that I was so cute and was rockin' my maternity swimsuit. Needless to say, it made my day. I would suspect that most pregnant woman don't feel as attractive as when they aren't pregnant, and they definitely need to hear that they are. Even if that bump is huge, just call it cute and let them know they look good pregnant.

3. "How far along are you?" The most important thing about this question is that there is no follow up as to size. But asking how far along they are invites a conversation with them and gives you a chance to say more nice things! But caution; make sure you ask it this way and not "How long do you have left?" I may have snapped at someone a little bit when they asked me that and I had a little over a week left. At that point, you just want that baby out and anyone is a target for your frustration.

4. "Are you having a boy or a girl?" This is a safe question to ask because it doesn't talk about size, and it gives you something exciting to talk about. Regardless of whether women know if it's a boy or a girl, they are going to be excited about the gender of their baby. So, let them talk about it! And congratulate them no matter what they are having. Boys and girls are both fun and you don't want to tell them how hard one of them is (because with all of those fun pregnancy emotions, you could easily upset them).

5. "How are you feeling?" Quite honestly, I just like to complain at the end of pregnancy. It's dang hard making a baby, and with all of my pregnancies, my body did not love me back. My poor husband got a lot of my complaints, but it would have been super nice if someone had asked me how I was feeling so I could just vent a little (and he probably would have appreciated it, too).

6. "Your bump is adorable!" Again, just make her feel good about her growing belly. Let her know she looks great, her bump is cute, and she is doing a great job.

Most importantly, don't say anything about size! If you aren't sure if it's an okay thing to ask, ask yourself if you would be referencing her size and then there's your answer. Good luck navigating the turbulent waters of talking to a pregnant woman!

Things You Can Blame on Pregnancy

Pregnancy is the ultimate excuse. There have been instances where my husband has told me he doesn't like when I'm pregnant because I seriously blame everything on pregnancy. But to be fair, making a baby is hard and it does a lot of weird and difficult stuff to your body.

Sometimes when you're pregnant there are things you just can't control, and you can always blame those things on being pregnant. Here are some things I have definitely blamed on pregnancy:

1. Cravings. I'm not talking about "Oh, I really want pizza" cravings here. I'm talking about wanting pizza so bad that it's all you can talk about and all you can think about. You want it so bad that until you get that specific food, you will not be satisfied. There were several times that I had to bribe my husband to go get something for me because I wanted it so bad. Like Pizza Hut breadsticks with cheese. Those things get me during pregnancy. And, lucky for you, you can just be like "I'm pregnant!" and then it justifies your cravings and people usually feel sympathetic enough to go get it for you. Suckers!

2. Wanting to eat all the time. Since you are growing a human, you are going to need about 300 extra calories per day. But somehow that translates into wanting to eat ALL THE TIME! And also wanting to eat at weird times. It's 3 a.m.? Your body doesn't care if you're sleeping, it wants food now. But just blame it on pregnancy and people will excuse your giant appetite.

3. Gas. When you have a person in your uterus it makes you super gassy. And because of that tiny person in your uterus it's a lot harder to hold that gas in. It's super unfortunate and kind of cruel, but it happens. And when you do let one slip, just blame it on pregnancy. Because it really is hard to hold it in when you are pregnant!

4. Nausea. If you tell someone you feel sick and then follow that up with "I'm pregnant," they'll be like "Ohhh, I'm so sorry! Is there anything I can do?" There probably isn't anything, but if you tell someone you are nauseous

because you are pregnant they'll definitely understand and be super nice in response. Sometimes it's all you can do to just sit and try not to think about how sick you feel, and it sucks. So, yes, just blame it on pregnancy.

5. Sleeping a lot. I don't mean getting a good solid eight hours. I mean sleeping ten hours during the night, and then napping at random times throughout the day. There were several times I fell asleep watching my kids play when I was pregnant with my third baby. I would just blame it on pregnancy and it made me feel at least a little bit better. And when your husband complains that you want to go to bed at 9 p.m., just blame it on pregnancy and tell him goodnight.

6. Laziness. Is the TV remote out of your reach? Well when you're pregnant, sometimes that is just too far. You're either too nauseous to move, too sore to move, or you have sunk too deep into your couch to be able to get up and get it yourself. So, while some people might call it laziness, you know better. It's because of pregnancy.

7. Soreness. You get to a point in pregnancy where your whole body hurts. Your ribs are killing you, it hurts to walk because your hips are being stretched out, your lower back hurts, and even your feet feel like you've walked a million miles (even if you haven't left the house). Having a human in your belly makes your body stretch and, of course, that's going to make things a bit painful. Hence, the famous pregnancy waddle.

8. Peeing all the time. In the first trimester, you are peeing all the time because hormonal changes fill your bladder more often, not to mention the increase in blood leads to extra fluid being processed in your kidneys; hence, having to pee more. And then in the third trimester your baby is

pushing right on that bladder making you have to pee more. Good luck going on a road trip when you are pregnant because you are going to be stopping ALL THE TIME, even if you aren't drinking a lot (which you still should because you're pregnant). So, when your family or friends sigh and say, "Again?" when you get up, just blame it on pregnancy.

Lots of crazy things happen to your pregnant body that you can't control but, luckily, you can just tell people "It's because I'm pregnant" and they'll hopefully understand. Being pregnant can be hard, but it's so worth it in the end. So, enjoy using that excuse because soon you won't be able to blame that midnight fourth meal run to Taco Bell on pregnancy.

The "H" Word

I've already mentioned it a few times, but I'm going to be straightforward with you and spill all the juicy details (maybe juicy isn't the right word...yuck). HEMORRHOIDS.

The first-time pregnant mom might be asking, "What's the big deal?" And if you're on your second or third pregnancy, you will most likely be nodding your head with tears in your eyes like "I feel ya, girl."

Hemorrhoids are basically varicose veins in your rectum. Sound gross? It is. And incredibly painful. If you get them, it's probably going to be in the third trimester, and it's going to make pooping a nightmare. Lots of fiber, lots of water, and stool softeners will help prevent constipation, but it still might hurt even when you aren't going to the bathroom.

Thank goodness for Preparation H, witch hazel pads, and pillows you can sit on.

Vulvar Varicosities

If you thought hemorrhoids were bad, you'll be horrified by these. If you have varicose veins in your legs, you might have these in your future. One study I read estimated that between 18-22% of pregnant women get them[1], but I have NEVER heard another woman confess to having these. To be fair, this is the first time I'm confessing to having them (it's all for the greater good). I think every woman should know how common they are and that there are ways to treat them.

Basically, vulvar varicosities are varicose veins in your vulva. They make your lady parts all swollen, look absolutely terrifying, and make sitting on any type of hard surface incredibly uncomfortable. Vulvar varicosities also make it hard to walk, sit, or stand for very long (so you're basically screwed if you get these). If we're being honest, I think they are my absolute least favorite thing I have ever experienced during all three of my pregnancies.

They didn't develop until the end of my third pregnancy, and they got progressively worse until delivery. I had to sit on pillows around the house, I couldn't walk very long without being incredibly sore the next day, and I couldn't sit on the floor and play with my kids. It was rough.

My doctor recommended getting a "support garment," which was basically like a really awkward lady jock strap. And as much as I hated wearing it, it really did make a difference. And lucky for me, the vulvar varicosities didn't cause any problems with delivery (which I was worried about), and they went away within a few days of my son's birth.

So, if you do end up getting them, they suck, I'm sorry, and know that you aren't alone (even if nobody EVER talks about them!).

Maternity Photos

I've only had maternity photos taken once, but I would 100% recommend it to every pregnant woman. Pregnancy is such a uniquely beautiful part of life, and after your baby is born it's really special to have pictures to look back at and see the amazing changes your body was going through.

Even if you aren't someone who is very comfortable in front of the camera, step outside of your comfort zone and do it. You won't regret it, and getting all dressed up and fancy will help boost your pregnant ego!

Own That Weight Gain

Pregnancy may be the only time in your life when you confidently step on the scale at the doctor's office and proudly pat your large belly. Any other time it's like "I gained three pounds in four weeks? Yikes!" But during pregnancy, it's like "GROW, BABY, GROW!" And towards the end of pregnancy that number will go up quicker. You might gain a pound (or two) a week in the third trimester![2] It's crazy, and definitely a unique thing to experience. So, own that weight gain, don't feel bad about it in the slightest, and enjoy the amazing things your growing body is doing.

Pregnancy Dreams

Dreams during pregnancy are about 1,000 times weirder than dreams when you aren't pregnant. That may not be a scientific fact, but it certainly feels like it. And not only are your dreams weird when you're pregnant, but you tend to remember them more clearly. When I was pregnant, I could recall dreaming almost every night!

There are lots of theories as to why this happens, but a combination of disrupted sleeping patterns (thanks, bladder), hormones, and changes in your emotional, mental, and physical state[3] (duh) are probably all to blame. Pregnancy impacts your entire body whether you're awake or asleep. If you can remember to do it, try writing down a few of your weird dreams when you wake up in the morning. Hopefully, you aren't having nightmares and, hopefully, your dreams are just happy or weird and not scary! Just know that it's normal, you aren't alone, and that this too shall pass.

Tips for Sleeping Better During Pregnancy

Speaking of sleeping and all of those crazy dreams, let's talk about sleeping during the third trimester. It's the WORST. I don't know about you, but I think that during pregnancy there are some nights when I get less sleep than when I have a newborn to feed every two hours. Between the back pain, the congestion, the heartburn, the hip pain, and having to go to the bathroom every hour, getting a good night's sleep during pregnancy can seem elusive.

It doesn't matter if you are on your first and have no other kids at home, or you're on your third pregnancy and have two other kids at home, if you don't get a good night's sleep, you probably will be a little bit of a hot mess the next day (I'm pretty sure my husband and kids can attest to that). And I also know that if I don't get a good night's sleep, my husband doesn't either, which is a big bummer because he often has to wake up super early for work every day.

Of course, there are some things you can't control, but there are lots of things you can do to help manage specific pregnancy sleeping problems. Here are some helpful tips for sleeping better during pregnancy:

1. Don't drink anything after dinner. One common problem pregnant women experience is waking up to pee at night. I've found that on nights that I drink any water or juice after dinner, I usually have to get up and go to the bathroom a lot. So limit yourself and just don't drink anything after dinner. I would suggest not drinking anything after 7 p.m., because that gives you a few hours to get whatever you drank earlier out of your system before climbing into bed. And that way, you will have to get up fewer times in the night! Yay!

2. Don't drink caffeine in the evening. There are a lot of conflicting studies about caffeine during pregnancy, but experts recommend limiting your total daily caffeine consumption to less than 200 mg[4]. And if you are a caffeine drinker and need that little extra boost to help you get through the day, just make sure you aren't drinking it in the evening. Caffeine increases the frequency of urination and it can increase your heart rate, both of which are not conducive to sleeping. So, just try to get your caffeine fix earlier in the day if you need it!

3. Don't work out at night. This goes for anybody, but especially a pregnant woman. Have you ever gone for a jog or played basketball or done some cardio after the kids

have gone to bed? Were you able to get to sleep on time? My husband used to play basketball in the evenings sometimes and, every single time, he had a hard time falling asleep. Your body gets stimulated when you exercise, and obviously that's a bad thing if you're planning on falling asleep soon after. So, even though exercise is definitely an important part of pregnancy, try to do it earlier in the day so you can sleep better at night.

4. Use nasal strips to help with congestion. During pregnancy my nighttime congestion is off the charts. I was curious why so during my first pregnancy I looked it up and found out that congestion during pregnancy is very common! And if you don't want to be up all night with a clogged nose or keeping your husband up all night with your loud open-mouth breathing, try using nasal strips to help with congestion. In our family, congestion is probably the biggest pregnancy problem that keeps my husband up at night, so the nights when my congestion is bad, my nasal strips really make a difference in the quality of our sleep!

5. Do something relaxing before bed. There are lots of things you can do to relax such as meditation, listening to affirmations, journaling, reading, or listening to calming music in a dimly-lit bedroom. If you feel stressed or have a hard time turning your brain off (me!), then doing something to help relax you before bed is a great way to help your mind calm down and help you fall asleep faster. Pregnancy comes with a lot of thoughts and feelings, and if you don't find a way to deal with that stress, you're probably going to have a hard time sleeping.

6. Take a warm bath or shower before bed. Since I usually don't get a lot of time to myself in the mornings, I like to shower at night after the kids are in bed. Not only does it

help me feel clean and refreshed before bed, but it helps relax my muscles and ease any aches I have. Pregnancy is hard on your body, and taking a warm bath or shower really helps alleviate some of that pain. I don't know about you, but body aches and pains are one thing that keep me from having a good night's sleep during pregnancy, and when I take a warm shower before bed I usually sleep better!

7. Sleep with pillows between your legs and under your belly. This is one of the most important things I do to help myself sleep better. Since you're supposed to sleep on your side during pregnancy, and that's definitely not always the comfiest position, sleeping with some support between your knees and calves and under your belly can really help you feel more comfortable. Personally, it helps my hips not hurt as much at night, too. Sometimes I even sleep with a pillow behind my back to give me some extra support. I know you can buy a fancy pregnancy pillow to help with this, but you really don't need to if you have extra pillows already on your bed. And even though it takes a few adjustments for me to switch positions at night (because rolling over in bed in the third trimester is an absolute joke), I'm usually so tired that I fall right back asleep and don't even wake my husband.

8. Wear comfy pajamas to bed. You might think this sound silly, but if you don't have on comfy pajamas when you sleep, you aren't going to be able to rest well, especially during pregnancy. I love wearing leggings and loose, soft tees to bed, and it really helps me sleep deeper because I don't have to adjust my clothes at night. It's just one more small thing you can do to help you sleep better during pregnancy.

9. Take antacids before bed. I was going to recommend not eating spicy or greasy food for dinner, but is that even possible? Curry, pizza, burgers, and Mexican food, get in my belly. So, yes, you could avoid spicy or greasy food in the evenings, or you could also just take some antacids before you go to bed at night when you do eat those things!

Hopefully these tips for sleeping better during pregnancy will be helpful if you're looking for a better night's sleep. My husband sleeps better when I do these things, too, and that definitely makes for better days for everyone at our house!

Seeing Your Entire Belly Move From the Outside

If you thought it was cool to feel your baby kick from the inside, just wait until he is so big that when he changes positions your entire belly moves!

I distinctly remember a time when I was super pregnant with my first baby and I was sitting in a women's meeting at church. I was listening to the teacher talk, and I looked down at my belly and saw the entire thing move a few centimeters to the left, and then back to the center. My eyes widened in surprise and I quickly looked around to see if anyone else had noticed. Of course, it was just me because nobody else had been watching my stomach, but I was amazed.

If you haven't experienced this movement yet, just wait, because it will probably blow your mind. Yes, you've seen your baby on an ultrasound and you've felt him move from the inside, but it's just another form of proof that there is a living, growing human inside your belly, and there really is nothing quite like it.

Pregnant Women Can't Do Anything Fun

I love sledding. I love sitting at the top of a big hill right before going down, I love feeling the sting of the cold air and snow blowing on my face as I rush down, and I love tumbling off the sled at the bottom of the hill when the ride is over.

Unfortunately, three of the last five winters I have been pregnant and unable to do anything fun. You can't sled, you can't ski, and you can't ice skate when you're pregnant. And it's not just winter fun, either. Pregnant women can't go on roller coasters, can't go on water slides, and can't roller skate. You probably won't be able to go on long hikes, and you also shouldn't ride a bike.

It sort of seems like getting pregnant sucks the fun out of a lot of things, especially outdoor activities. Yes, it's wonderful and there are things about being pregnant that are awesome, but don't expect to go rock climbing or learn how to surf for the next nine months. You're going to have to get your adrenaline rushes somewhere else, Mama.

Mommy Brain Already?

Chances are you've heard the phrase "mommy brain" at some point. And if you were so naïve as to think that it only applied to moms who have birthed their babies, you have another thing coming.

With each of my pregnancies, I have gotten progressively worse at remembering things. With my first baby, I quickly discovered that pregnancy made me incredibly forgetful, and if I didn't write something down, it wasn't going to happen. I was always asking my husband things multiple times until I actually wrote them down. And without a grocery list, I couldn't remember to buy even the simplest things, like milk or bread.

Pregnancy doesn't actually change your brain, but with new priorities, less quality sleep, and feelings of excitement, worry, and anticipation about your growing baby, you're probably going to find that you have more on your mind and it's harder to keep track of things.

Now that I have three kids, I absolutely have to write things down. I have become a list person who fills notebooks with all kinds of grocery lists, to-do lists, bucket lists, and shopping lists. I also have to have a planner to keep track of my family's schedule (and even then I still forget things). So, you might as well get used to it during pregnancy because mommy brain isn't going anywhere.

PMS That Lasts Nine Months

You know how when you're PMSing everything makes you cry? You might see a commercial for a window cleaner where the mom is constantly having to clean fingerprints and then one day, she realizes the windows are clean and you see that her kids are grown up and she misses the fingerprint-marked windows, and then you also realize that you are sobbing uncontrollably and can't stop? Pregnancy is like that but for nine months.

You cry super easily, you're extra sensitive, and the silliest things can get you worked up.

There's an episode of The Office where Pam is pregnant and she keeps sobbing over this commercial about a dog who wants to protect his bone, which if you watch the commercial it's really not one that would normally make you feel sad, but to a pregnant woman, it's super sad. I watch that episode when I'm pregnant and I am right there with her.

It's especially rough for anyone who interacts with you on a daily basis because they have to tread lightly and be careful with what they say because at any moment, you could snap and start crying or yelling.

In the third trimester, when everything hurts and you are just so done with being pregnant, you really have to be aware of your feelings. I remember I was 37 weeks with my daughter and one Sunday at church a kind lady innocently asked me, "You're still here, huh?" That poor woman. Yes, I looked like I could have my baby any day, but I did not want to be reminded that I still had a while left to go and I just lost it. I later apologized, but my irrational, emotional, pregnant self said some unkind things that were probably not so appropriate for church.

Pregnancy is beautiful, but it really is like PMS that lasts for nine months. And that sucks.

Counting Kicks

I still remember the bright yellow pamphlet that my OB gave me when I hit the six month mark. It had a big blue pregnant belly and a hand that was holding a stopwatch. I was so excited to start keeping track of how often my son moved every day and I immediately went home and tried it.

Most days I would feel him move ten times in a pretty short amount of time, and I liked the peace of mind that came with knowing that he was doing what he was "supposed " to be doing.

But by the end of pregnancy, I was so tired of counting kicks each day. Yes, it's important to make sure your baby is moving and following the same pattern so you can know if something is wrong, but eventually counting kicks stressed me out and I even had a false alarm and thought something was wrong when it wasn't.

Pay attention to your body and if you're aware of your baby's normal movement, you'll notice if something is off. And if you think it is, it's worth calling the doctor to make sure your baby is okay!

Dear Husband

Dear Sweet, Kind, Loving Husband,

I'm sorry. I'm sorry for all the complaining I do. I'm sorry for all the restless nights I spend in bed that keep you awake and eventually lead to you sleeping on the sofa. I'm sorry for not ever wanting to go anywhere because my entire body hurts. I'm sorry for pestering you to go get me a Doritos Locos Taco at 11pm, and then not being able to eat it when you got home because the smell made me nauseous. I'm sorry for the horrible gas that I can't hold in (especially on that one very long and stinky road trip). I'm sorry for using pregnancy as an excuse to get out of yard work, cleaning the house, vacuuming the car, and basically anything else I don't want to do.

Love,

Your Pregnant Wife

Pregnant Women Should do Hair Commercials

You know those old Herbal Essences commercials where the women had beautiful, thick hair that they whipped around them while shouting, "Yes, yes, yes!"?

That's how my hair looks during pregnancy. It's AMAZING.

During pregnancy, my hair grows fast, it doesn't fall out, it has more volume, it's shiny, and it just looks so healthy.

I seriously feel like if I went to go audition for a hair commercial, I could walk in with no acting experience (unless you count my role in my fifth grade class play about Marco Polo) and they would immediately give me the role. My amazing hair would compensate for my acting, no matter how awkward and unbelievable it was.

For real, if you are strapped for cash when you're pregnant and need to make some fast money, just go audition for a hair commercial. You will definitely get it. Hair like that doesn't grow on trees (it just grows on pregnant women and goddesses).

"Do You Have a Name Picked Out?"

There's one question that almost always follows after people ask what gender your baby is. They almost always ask, "Do you have a name picked out?"

It's an innocent question, and some people can give an answer immediately. Some people even know what they're going to name their baby, boy or girl, before they get pregnant.

Then there's my husband and me. Our first baby didn't get named until we were on the way to the hospital, and our second and third babies didn't get named until several hours after they were born. They were just "Baby" until we officially decided what to call them.

To be fair, naming your baby is a big deal. You are giving a person a name that will follow him or her around forever. It's definitely not something you should take lightly.

Looking at baby name books and lists online can be fun, but it's hard agreeing on a name. Your husband will like one name, but it will remind you of someone you knew whom you didn't like, so you can't go with that one. Then you'll like one and he'll tell you that he dated someone with that name and it will be forever ruined for you.

You don't want it to be a trendy name, and you don't want it to be a name that every other baby born that year will have. You don't want it to rhyme with anything bad or funny, and you don't want the baby's initials to spell out anything obscene.

And then, as if picking one name wasn't hard enough, you may want to pick a middle name that goes with the first name that you've chosen, too. And, unfortunately, some names, no matter how cute or beautiful they are on their own, just don't go together.

No matter what you decide to name your baby, there's always that one person who plasters on a fake smile and responds with, "Oh, that's nice," or "What a unique name," and you can tell they absolutely hate the name you've chosen but are just trying to be polite.

Naming a baby is hard, and whether you decide what to name your baby before you get pregnant or a few hours after they're born, it's okay. Just please don't name your child after a food (I'm looking at you, Gwyneth Paltrow).

Objects on Body Are Larger Than They May Appear

One thing you'll quickly discover as your pregnancy progresses is that your belly gets in the way pretty often.

There are times when you'll try and fit into a tight space and realize that you can't because your belly is in the way.

It might be in a busy crowd trying to squeeze between people, trying to close the door in a regular-sized bathroom stall, or trying to get out of your car after parking in a narrow space. You might not be able to fit in a crowded elevator or into booths when you go out to eat, and squeezing between rows at the movie theater can get awkward and uncomfortable for everyone.

Sometimes you just forget that your belly is as big as it is, and sometimes you forget to compensate. Sometimes you do try and compensate, and it's just not enough. Getting stuck or not fitting in tight places is definitely one of the times when you have to laugh to keep from crying (thanks again, hormones).

Fortunately, it doesn't last forever, and you'll be choosing regular stalls instead of the large stalls in no time.

Nesting (Because "Mad Desire to Deep Clean and Get Baby's Room Ready" Doesn't Sound as Cute)

Before I even start talking about how weird nesting is, let's quickly mention how weird the name is! I mean, I get that birds make nests to keep their little eggies safe and keep their babies safe from predators once they're born, but couldn't someone have come up with a better name?

Nesting usually hits towards the end of pregnancy, and this usually involves doing everything you can to get your home ready for your baby. Whether that involves sewing a quilt, crib sheet, curtains, and changing pad cover (like me), deep cleaning all of your carpets, or re-painting your entire home, the crazy desire to prepare for your new addition is real.

Your husband will probably think you're crazy when you're up at 2am drawing plans for how you want to decorate the nursery, and thank goodness for Pinterest so you can make a "vision board" and pin color schemes, décor, and bedding that you like (seriously, what would we do without Pinterest?).

And along with nesting comes a surge of energy to actually do all of these things you want to do, which is nice because it'll probably hit in the third trimester when your energy has started to go downhill again. Without that urge, you'd just be sitting on the couch staring around your home at all the things you'd like to fix and redecorate, and that's no good.

Once you feel like baby's room is ready, you'll probably still find other things to do, whether that's wash and hang up all of baby's clothes, clean out your car (even in the hard-to-clean spots you've been putting off for years), and reorganize every cabinet and drawer in your kitchen. It's exhausting, but also a great way to stay busy.

I mean, you might as well while you have the time and energy because once your baby comes, you know you're not going to even be thinking about cleaning behind your toilets.

Comfort? What's That?

You are never truly comfortable in the third trimester.

No matter what position you sit in, stand in, or lie in, there's pain somewhere. And if you think you might be about to get comfortable, your body will be like, "Nope, you have to pee," or your baby will move and his foot will be up under your ribs making it hard for you to breathe deeply. You'll try to drink less and wear yoga pants that won't put as much pressure on your belly. You'll try to massage your belly to get him to move (and sometimes you'll actually bend over and try telling him to move). But, Mama, it won't work, and you'll still be uncomfortable all the way up until he's born (and then a few days after).

The words "comfort" and "third trimester" just don't belong in the same sentence together. Sorry.

The Pregnant Shuffle

At first it might seem like a name for a hip new dance move, but nope. This, my friends, is what I call the way a pregnant woman moves during the last few weeks of pregnancy.

They say to try and "walk the baby out" to get labor going, but you have to weigh the pros and cons of getting up and walking around. Yes, it might get labor going, but it also might cause you to be the source of endless ridicule from family and friends.

My husband loves to make fun of how slow I move and how I can barely even waddle at the end of pregnancy. I can hardly keep up with him when we go places together and I am constantly asking him to slow down. I pretty much shuffle around like an 80-year-old in a robe and house slippers those last few weeks of pregnancy. It's rough.

Maybe we should band together and make it a cool new dance move to make it seem like we're doing it on purpose? No? Okay, maybe next time.

When You Gotta Go

Peeing in the third trimester is especially rough. Your baby will move a little bit and you'll be like, "I HAVE TO PEE NOW." And then if you don't find a bathroom immediately, the world feels like it's going to end. Then, once you do go, only an ounce comes out (we're talking not even enough to fill one of those tiny Dixie cups) and you'll be like "ARE YOU KIDDING ME?" And you'll have the pleasure of going through this cycle about 50 times a day because that's super fun. Everyone in your family will hate going places with you because you spend half the time you're out looking for the closest bathroom. Like I said, it's rough.

Are Those My Ankles or an Elephant's Ankles?

Ever heard of cankles? They sound funny until you get them yourself. At the end of pregnancy, your feet and ankles will probably swell a little bit, especially if you're on your feet a lot; and if it gets bad, it might look like your ankles disappear and your calf goes straight down to your foot resulting in calf-ankles or cankles.

I thought that I had bad cankles with my third baby until I saw my sister's cankles. Becca, I'm sorry, but I had a really good laugh when I saw what pregnancy did to your ankles (thanks for that, by the way). But to be fair, you're a teacher and basically spent all day on your feet right up until delivery. Bless you, child, bless you.

Cankles are kind of a mean way to describe it, but at least it's a descriptive term. I always think about how elephants don't have ankles and their legs just go straight down to their feet. That's how I picture pregnant women's ankles (or lack of ankles).

If you get bad cankles, try and rest, elevate your feet, and try wearing some compression stockings. Your ankles might be ugly for a while, but at least they'll go back to normal within a few days after delivery (sorry, elephants, but you're stuck with cankles forever).

The Baby Shower

During the course of my three pregnancies, I've had four baby showers. With my first pregnancy, my mom and sister threw one for me in my hometown, and then my friends threw one for my best friend and I (because we were due two weeks apart) where we lived in Iowa. With my second pregnancy, my friends threw me a diaper shower (which is slightly different, but not really) since I had most of what I already needed. With my third pregnancy, my friends threw me a baby shower and gave me some basics (diapers, baby lotion, etc.) as well as a few new outfits for little man since he was the second boy and destined to wear hand-me-downs his whole life.

Baby showers are a great way to get things you might need, and they're a great excuse to eat dessert (I'm only sort of kidding with that last bit because who doesn't need more cake in her life?). And if a formal shower isn't your thing, ask a few lady friends to go out to brunch with you and celebrate that way.

Whether it's your first pregnancy or your third, have a shower. Every pregnant mom deserves to be celebrated, even if it's not her first baby. You're still carrying that baby around for nine months and you deserve to be treated!

What to Put on Your Baby Registry

The first time your pregnant self walks into the baby store can be crazy overwhelming. So many brands, so many things that people say you MUST buy, so many things you have no idea how to use (or why you would even use them). It's hard to know what is actually helpful and what is a waste of money when it comes to baby products. Especially because some of them can be expensive!

One of the best ways to get some of those pricier items is to add them to your baby registry! You never know who is going to be super generous, or if your coworkers might want to chip in and buy you that fancy stroller you have your eye on. And you can often get coupons or discounts to buy things that people don't purchase after your baby is born!

Here are some helpful suggestions of things to add to your baby registry:

1. A car seat. You're going to have to get one of these anyway, so you might as well add it to your registry!

2. Portable crib (like a pack n' play). We have used our portable crib for vacations, camping, naps at home when the nursery is occupied or inaccessible, and as a playpen outside. There are lots of different styles of portable cribs, and some of them even have changing pads or bassinets attached. I highly recommend getting one because these things are pretty much essential.

3. Baby monitor. We've done regular audio monitors and video monitors, and while both are great, I love the peace of mind of having a video monitor to check on my baby. It's not an absolute essential, but it does make a big difference in easing your stressed-out mommy mind, and you can use them for years (we still have one in our big kids' room).

4. Stroller. Whether you register for a stroller that matches your car seat, or a fancier one that can eventually convert to a double stroller, adding a stroller to your registry is a great idea. I can guarantee you're going to want one of these bad boys, even if you just use it for mom walks around the mall.

5. Bouncer, swing, or jumper. We've used all of these with our kids, and they have come in handy a lot! When your baby is a newborn, the bouncer is a great place to set them when you have your hands full and want to keep

them close. Swings are helpful when you can't get baby to calm down and are close to a mental breakdown. And our jumper has easily been one of our favorite baby items as our babies have gotten a bit bigger. They've all loved hanging out in that thing!

6. Baby clothes. People are going to get you these anyway, so it's nice to register for a few things so people have an idea of your style! You'll need some sleepers, baby socks and mittens, a hat, bodysuits, and some little pants. And register for things in different sizes!

7. Healthcare and grooming kit. One of my favorite (and one of the most helpful) things we got off of our baby registry was a baby healthcare and grooming kit. I know it sounds weird, but it has things like a baby thermometer, nail clippers, nasal aspirator, medicine dispenser, and a comb. We've used it so many times and, seriously guys, it has been so helpful. I highly recommend adding one of these to your baby registry (and props to my sister who bought ours for us!).

8. Swaddle blanket. Swaddle blankets can be simple or fancy, and they range in price quite a bit. Having at least one is essential because that's how babies sleep at first! I can't imagine newborn life without a swaddle blanket.

9. Nursing pillow. A nursing pillow is so much more than just a regular pillow. Ladies, if you are planning to breastfeed, I insist you register for one of these. It makes all the difference in holding and positioning your baby, and in saving your back!

10. Diaper bag. Pick out one you like and add it to your registry! I've gone through several different styles of diaper bags (I currently love backpack ones so I can have

a baby on my hip and toddlers holding my hand). Yes, you can use a purse if you really want to, but I love all the different pockets, zippers, and space that diaper bags have!

11. White bodysuits. You can never have enough white bodysuits. They're one thing you can always have more of, and you need them in essentially every size! Babies are messy, and I can guarantee you're going to go through a lot of these. Add them to your registry and save yourself some money!

12. Baby carrier/wrap. I've tried four different baby carriers, and there are things I like and dislike about each. You might opt for one that straps onto your chest where your baby can be facing you or facing out, or you might be more of a wrap mama who likes to wear her baby around the house all day long. Do your research, pick one, and add it to your registry.

13. Bumbo. I've used our Bumbo seat for all three kids and I love it. We've used it for learning how to sit, feeding, and even just hanging out in! They are super sturdy and will last through multiple kids, so I highly suggest getting one with your first baby!

14. Baby memory book. I know that some people don't use baby books anymore, but I love having a place to write down the new things my babies do each month, their first words, what things were like when they were born, and their growth percentiles. I even have my own baby book from when I was a baby! You should consider getting a memory book because they're a great way to record memories, doctor's visits, and important milestones. And adding it to your baby registry is a great way to get one for free!

15. Bathtub. It's not a necessity because you can easily just roll a towel up under baby's head and do a very low water level, but if you want to have a baby bathtub, add it to your registry!

16. Books. Can a child ever have too many books? You can register for certain books if there are ones you love and want for your child, or you can even have guests bring books to the shower in lieu of cards. It's never too early to start reading to your baby!

17. Diapers. Duh.

18. Wipes. Again, duh.

19. Diaper rash cream. Important to have on hand before you actually need it. You don't want to open up a diaper one day to find a furious, red rash and not have any diaper cream to treat it!

20. A diaper pail. Not a necessity because you can just throw diapers away in the garage, but I've loved having one for my third baby, especially because our daughter has also been in diapers the whole time he's been alive!

21. Baby wash and lotion. Babies have sensitive skin so you need products that are just for them, and also, they smell amazing!

22. A high chair. No, you're not going to need this for a while, but you might as well register for one!

23. Burp rags and bibs. You never know if your baby is going to be a drooler or spitter, so it's nice to have a few handy just in case.

What Not to Put on Your Baby Registry

There are lots of lists online of things you have to put on your baby registry. Most of the time, the authors claim that they just can't live without the things on their list and that those things have changed their lives and made parenting sooo much easier. Things that might be cute or sound like a good idea, but that aren't very functional, are completely unnecessary, or that you can get along without just fine are often on their lists. After three kids, I think I know a thing or two about what baby items you actually need, and what baby items you don't need. Here are five things you definitely should not put on your baby registry:

1. A wipe warmer. I see the appeal of these and, yes, I did use one for a while with my first baby, but they are so unnecessary. It's not mean to use a room-temperature wipe on your baby's bum, and they will be fine if the wipes you are using aren't warmed up. Do you warm up your toilet paper? No, because that would be weird. Don't buy a wipe warmer.

2. Baby shoes. Guys, just don't. They are so unnecessary. They might look cute, but they're a waste of money (says the girl who bought two pairs of baby Nikes for her son that he almost NEVER wore). Plus their feet grow so dang fast that they only get to wear them a few times anyway. And honestly, you don't need shoes if you're not walking!

3. A bottle sterilizer or bottle warmer. Ladies, don't waste your money on something dish soap and hot water from the microwave can do.

4. A baby Keurig. The most ridiculous baby item I have ever seen that you absolutely do not need is a machine that is like a Keurig but makes bottles of formula. You really

can't just scoop it and shake it yourself? I officially look down on you if you buy one of these. Shame.

5. A baby food maker. I get it if you want to make your own baby food, but just use a blender or food processor. That's basically all a baby food maker is. Don't go spend money on something you probably already have just because it has the name "baby" in it.

Be smart about what you buy for your baby, don't get overwhelmed, and use common sense when you are preparing. And if one of these things on this list is something you still want, then by all means go for it. Unless it's the baby Keurig. Never, ever buy that.

Staying in Bed All Day Isn't Actually as Fun as it Sounds

I have been incredibly fortunate during all three of my pregnancies and have never had to be put on bed rest. But best rest is actually pretty common (especially when you're pregnant with multiples).

Since I don't have any personal experience with bed rest, I talked to a few of my friends who have been put on bed rest, whether because of twin pregnancies, incompetent cervix, preeclampsia, premature labor, or for something else. From what I've heard, it is far from relaxing.

It might sound fun at first to relax and watch Netflix all day, but it can get old pretty quickly. Your muscles might atrophy (depending on how long you have to be on bed rest), you may have to ask for help from friends and family to bring meals, get groceries, and clean your home, and you'll probably have to try out some new hobbies that don't involve moving around (like knitting, painting, or puzzles).

It's especially hard if you have a full-time (or even part-time) job or you're going to school because you really have to scale back and find a way to make it work, or take some time off. The health of your baby is the most important thing and, unfortunately, other people don't always understand that.

If you get put on bed rest, I'm sorry. It sucks, it's hard, and it's definitely boring. Just remember why you're doing it, take it seriously, and know you're not alone. And if it helps keep your baby cooking a little longer, it is 110% worth it.

Questions to Ask on a Hospital Tour

Before our first baby was born my husband and I took a maternity hospital tour to see where we would be staying and where our baby would be born. It was really helpful in preparing me for our son's birth. Our second son was born in a different hospital in a different state, so even though he was our third baby and I had a pretty good idea about what to expect, I still went and did another hospital tour.

Taking a hospital tour gives you a chance to ask any questions you might have about what the hospital offers, what they allow, and what childbirth there is like. It's a good idea for any mother who will be delivering there for the first time. If you're not sure what kinds of questions to ask on your hospital tour, here are some that you might want to know. Keep in mind that a lot of these will be answered by your tour guide (usually a L&D nurse), and some of them may not apply to you.

Preggers

Can I wear my own hospital gown?

Can I have a photographer take photos during the birth?

Can I have a photographer take photos after the birth?

Can I have a photographer take photos if I need to have a C-section?

What kind of pain management options do you have available (epidural, spinal block, tub, shower, IV, local anesthesia)?

Can my doula attend the birth?

Does the hospital support natural births?

What kind of birthing tools are available (tub, shower, birth ball, squat bar, birthing stool)?

How many rooms are on the labor and delivery floor?

Where is the best place to park when I arrive?

Where do I go when I arrive?

What do I need to bring?

Can I pre-register?

Are the delivery rooms private or are they shared?

Are the recovery rooms private or are they shared?

Are the rooms all the same size, and do they have the same features?

What happens if the labor and delivery floor is full and I'm in active labor?

Is this a teaching hospital?

Will students or residents attend the birth?

Are meals provided for me after birth?

Are meals provided for the father after the birth?

Can the father sleep at the hospital?

Is there a nursery for the baby to go to at night?

Where is the nursery?

Where is the NICU?

What level is the NICU and what is the youngest gestational age of baby they care for?

What kind of fetal and maternal monitoring is used?

How often do you do pelvic exams during labor?

Can I have music?

Is there a speaker in the room or do I need to bring my own?

How many people are allowed in the delivery room?

What positions do you allow mothers to give birth in (stirrups on back, in tub, on all fours, sitting up, squatting)?

Can we do skin-to-skin right after the baby is born and delay procedures and weighing?

Can I breastfeed immediately after delivery?

What kind of breastfeeding support is available?

Do you give pacifiers to babies in the nursery?

Do you give formula to babies in the nursery?

What kind of security measures do you have in place?

When are visiting hours?

Can children come visit?

How long do moms typically stay after birth?

Where will I be initially examined upon arriving (own room or triage)?

Can I walk around during labor?

Can I labor in the shower or tub?

Will I be moved to a room postpartum or stay in the same room?

Are there televisions?

Are there DVD players?

Is there Wi-Fi?

Can my husband (or baby's father) cut the cord?

Is there a private shower in the recovery room?

What is the hospital's C-section rate?

What happens if I need an emergency C-section?

Is there a hospital cafeteria? Is it open 24 hours?

Can I eat or drink during labor?

What kinds of things are provided for the baby?

What can I take home from the hospital with me (diapers, wipes, maxi pads)?

I know that's a lot of questions, but your tour guide will answer a lot of them before you even ask them, and some questions might not apply to you. Taking a hospital tour when you're pregnant is incredibly helpful and will make you feel so much more comfortable when it's go time. And preparing questions to ask on your hospital tour before you go will help you get the most out of your tour! Good luck!

Things to Do Before Your Baby is Born

I've already mentioned that my forgetfulness has made me a list person, but I am very big on lists. I make grocery lists, to-do lists, lists of things I want to buy, and lists of things I want to make. So, needless to say, I had a whole big list of things to do while I was pregnant before my first baby was born. It was super helpful because not only did it keep me busy until he got here, but the things I did were things that helped me out once he was born, too. I wasn't rushing around trying to get addresses for announcements or worrying about little things like what we were going to have for dinner once we got home. I was able to relax and enjoy the time with our new bundle of joy because I had planned things beforehand.

I originally posted a list of 25 things on my blog, but then I remembered more things I did and posted those, too. So this list has 40 things to do before your baby is born that will help make birth and the transition to parenthood easier and more enjoyable for you! Even though I personally did all of these, they aren't all for everyone, and I will not be offended if you don't add something to your list. So, grab a pen and start copying some of these down for your own list!

1. Pick a birth announcement. If you live far from family and friends, or if you just want to show off your perfect new baby (Who doesn't want that?), a birth announcement is a great way to introduce your newborn. You can either do something simple yourself by copying something online, or you can use a photo website with premade layouts. If you've already decided what you want before your baby is born, you won't have to stress about picking a birth announcement after they're born.

2. Gather addresses. If you decide you want to send out birth announcements, it can be even more stressful to gather all the addresses and figure out who you want to send them to after your baby is born. So, do it before! You

can compile them all into a Word document with a label template and print them out while you are pregnant so that when you get your announcements, you just have to put the sticky labels on the envelopes and send them away. Plus, if you work on it while you are pregnant you can have time to think about who you want to send them to and you'll know how many to order when the time comes!

3. Get a waterproof bed pad. Not for baby, for you. My husband and I had a nice pillow-top mattress that my parents bought us when we got married, and I was not about to have my water break on it and ruin it (even though we have replaced it now). I was worried that if my water did break in the middle of the night, we would have to leave fast and the amniotic fluid would do some seriously gross damage to our mattress while we were away at the hospital. So, instead of being nervous to fall asleep as your due date approaches, invest in a waterproof bed pad (search "waterproof mattress protector" online) that you can just put under the sheets on your side of the bed. And don't try and be cheap and think you can get one of those plastic drop cloths that you use for painting. I tried that on top of our mattress at first and it made way too much noise for me to even be able to fall asleep. Which, at that point in your pregnancy, you need to try and get as much sleep as you can between the ten bathroom trips each night. And even if your water doesn't break until you are at the hospital (like me), it's better to be safe than sorry!

4. Pack your bags. Since you never know when baby is going to come, the sooner the better with this one. You should pack a bag for you, a bag for baby, and if your husband is smart, he will let you pack a little bag for him (lists on what to pack are coming up). I had my bags packed and sitting by the front door a month before my

due date every single pregnancy. Yes, I was excited, but I was also prepared and had everything I needed at the hospital!

5. Get your carpets cleaned. Now this may not be appropriate for everyone, but living in an apartment that has nasty carpet and weird stains from the previous tenants made me really want to get our carpets cleaned. So, about a month before my due date with our first baby I rented a carpet cleaner and cleaned our carpets. Not only did they smell amazing and feel way softer after, I felt much better about our son rolling around on the floor. Plus, if you haven't done this in a while, it might be a nice thing to do before baby is born because after birth, you are not going to have time to do this. I also did a Google search for some coupons and called around at a few stores to get the best deal. You definitely will want to look into that.

6. Pick a doctor for your baby. If you don't have a family doctor or pediatrician for older children (or if you don't have older children and, therefore, no pediatrician), now is a good time to look for a doctor. Ask friends, look online at websites like healthgrades.com (but be cautious of how many people have reviewed them), and see if your hospital has contracts with any local offices. It's much easier to have this done before you have your baby because you don't want to be at the hospital holding your perfect little baby and have a minor panic attack when the nurse asks you who your baby's doctor is and tells you how soon you need to schedule your first appointment. Having a doctor picked out prior to your baby's birth is nice because you can go home and immediately schedule your baby's appointment without worrying about if you are calling a good doctor. Some doctors will let you come meet with them while you are pregnant for a kind of "meet

and greet" appointment. I did this the month before my first baby was born and the doctor I chose was the best pediatrician I've ever met (even after we've lived in three other states and have tried a bunch of pediatricians). So, it's definitely worth looking into. You also don't want to get to your first appointment and find out your doctor is not very friendly and doesn't have patience with your many questions from your first week home. No, thank you.

7. Pre-wash baby's clothes. Again, this is something you don't have to do and which won't be for everyone, but I wanted to make sure that all of my kids' clothes would be ready to go and not smell like the store. It was really fun to wash, fold, and put away all of those tiny clothes. And, yes, sometimes I would go and just smell the clothes in my babies' closets. It's just nice to have all of the clothes washed and put away before baby is born, especially if a lot of baby's clothes are from consignment sales or hand-me-downs from friends.

8. Invest in a nursing bra (or two). If you decide you are going to nurse your little baby, you will want to get a few nursing bras. You aren't supposed to use underwire until you've been breastfeeding for three months, and I personally like ones without underwire because I can use them when I'm sleeping and still be comfy. I would definitely recommend getting at least one nursing bra because trying to put nursing pads in a regular bra and moving it up all the time when you feed baby is pretty tough. It's a lot easier to have a nursing bra that clips and makes everything quickly accessible for when your baby is screaming because he's hungry. You can of course do this after baby is born, but it's nice to be able to bring a nursing bra to the hospital and wear it starting that first day.

9. Check to see if your insurance covers a breast pump. If you're going to nurse your baby, a breast pump is really nice to have for the times that you won't be able to nurse baby, or for when baby decides to sleep through the night and you wake up engorged and crying in pain because you have two rock-hard lumps on your chest. This particular point was very important for me because the hospital called and got the wrong information from someone at my insurance, and after being told it was covered, we got the fancy breast pump, only to find out four months later that it was not covered at all and we owed about $300. I know that since our first baby was born things have changed with insurance and breast pumps, but since I still have my original pump I've never had to worry about that. I would recommend calling (maybe even a few times to verify information) to see if your insurance covers a breast pump. It's really not fun to get a large bill later. And trust me, you will want at least some kind of breast pump. You never know how your baby is going to feed.

10. Make freezer meals. I was lucky during my first pregnancy because my best friend was due two weeks before me (Our boys are still best friends five years later!). We got together a month before my due date and made a ton of freezer meals. It's fun because it can take one day or it can take a few days (and when you are getting close to your due date you want to keep yourself busy). Just search online for freezer meals and you will have recipes galore. My husband and I found out that the recipes that we liked most were actually not crockpot ones, but ones that were casserole-like and were baked in the oven. Lasagna, pasta, and chicken fajitas were our personal favorites. And making freezer meals is really nice for after baby is born because once your family goes back home and you're left alone, the last thing you want to do is make a hot meal for you and your husband. After two days of

making freezer meals, our tiny freezer had almost no room for anything else. But it was so worth it, and was a huge help once our son was born (and if cooking's not your jam, just go buy some frozen dinners from the store!).

11. Attend classes at your hospital. Most hospitals offer free baby classes for expectant parents. I would highly recommend checking to see what kinds of classes you can take. My husband and I signed up for three, and even though he only went to one and I only went to two, it was really helpful. I took a notebook and filled up multiple pages with things like how to give baby a bath, how to care for a circumcision, breastfeeding tips, how to swaddle baby, and how to change a diaper (somehow I made it through life without changing a single diaper until my first baby was born). Plus, you can ask the teachers/nurses any additional questions you might have.

12. Install baby's car seat. I seriously think I drove around for about five weeks with my first baby's empty car seat in the backseat of my car before he was born. It's not super hard to do, but you don't want to get to the hospital and realize that you left your new baby's ride at home. A lot of police or fire stations will offer car seat installation checks where you can bring your car in and they will check to make sure you've installed the car seat correctly (Just make sure you call ahead to confirm they have someone working who is trained to check car seats.). Even if you've put a car seat in before, it's still a good idea to go have it checked out by a professional car seat checker. And when we got our convertible car seat a few months later, I took that in to get checked, too. It's always better to be safe than sorry.

13. Bake cookies to thank your nurses. Yes, this is sort of a silly one, but those nurses work hard and it's a nice

gesture! This obviously shouldn't be done until pretty close to your due date, but it is really nice to have a bag of cookies that you can give to the nurses once you are officially checked into the hospital. And if more than a few days goes by and you aren't in labor, it's always nice to have a bag of cookies waiting for you to make you feel better. You can make more for the nurses after you eat the first batch!

14. Get two waterproof mattress pads for the crib. I think most people probably only have one waterproof mattress pad on their crib, but I am clever and layered a waterproof mattress pad and then a fitted sheet, and then another mattress pad and another fitted sheet. That way, when my baby leaks through his diaper or throws up in the middle of the night, I can just pull the first layer off and he still has another protective layer there in case it happens again. You don't want to be trying to wash and put on a new mattress pad and sheet in the middle of the night. This has come in handy a few times for me, and it's definitely worth the extra bit of money to have a spare mattress pad on the bed (you'll thank me in the middle of the night).

15. Paint your nails. This may seem silly, too, but since you won't be feeling too glamorous after having a baby, it's nice to have your nails done to make you feel a little more put together! I painted my nails a nice baby blue color (since I was having a boy, duh) and it actually turned out really nice for the pictures that we had taken at the hospital. Plus, once your baby is born you are not going to have time to paint them and let them dry (especially if it's a color that needs two coats). Nope.

16. Buy some "in-between" clothes. One of my friends actually suggested this and I didn't do it during my first pregnancy and I regretted it. As much as you want your

pre-baby body back after your baby is born, it will not happen immediately. And since you won't be pregnant anymore, your emotional, postpartum self will not want to wear your maternity clothes. So before you have your baby, go buy some "in-between" clothes that you can wear until you fit back into your regular clothes. I'm never able to fit into my regular pants until a few months after my babies are born, and without a large, round belly, the band on your maternity pants is all saggy and you feel dumb wearing them. So, before you have your baby, just get a pair or two of in-between pants and maybe a few looser-fitting tops.

17. Look through your baby's baby book. If you haven't gotten a baby book, I highly recommend it. There are usually sections you can fill out before your baby is born about you and your husband, the day you found out you were pregnant, the ultrasound, the baby shower, and other things like that. Plus, you can see if there is a spot for a newspaper clipping from the day they are born and baby hand and footprints. Otherwise, you might not remember to get a newspaper or baby's footprints in the actual baby book. It also gives you all the feels to see the pages that talk about baby's birth and you will cry and be excited and scared and thrilled all at the same time while looking through them.

18. Charge your camera battery. Yes, I know that nearly everyone has a smart phone that can take pictures, but it's a good idea to bring your camera with a full battery to the hospital, especially if you have a nice DSLR. It was nice to be able to have my phone as a backup rather than my only way to take pictures. Plus, you will be taking like a million pictures at the hospital of your perfect new baby so you want to make sure your camera battery will last.

19. Do a test run to the hospital. If this is your first baby, or you haven't delivered at the hospital you are planning on having your baby at, it's a good idea to do a test run and see not only how long it takes you to get there, but to make sure you know exactly where to park and go once you have arrived. The signs outside of the hospitals we delivered at weren't super clear and it was nice to go and make sure we knew where to park, where to go in, what floor to go to, etc. Once you are in labor, you won't want to waste any time trying to figure that out.

20. Stock up on hand sanitizer. It's always nice to have some available for people to use before holding your baby, especially right after they're born and before they have immunizations. Having a doctor as a husband made me want to keep baby healthy even more (thanks for the worries, babe). It's always a good idea to try to keep your baby healthy.

21. Make your birth plan. You can write down things such as how you want your labor to go, what you want to do during labor, who you want in the room with you when baby is born, and if you want the chance to breastfeed right after baby is born (I'll give you more ideas in a few pages!). A birth plan is a really handy tool to have, and it can help put your mind at ease about delivery, even if you don't completely stick to it during labor (I'll talk more about this in a bit!).

22. Get a special notebook and folder for baby things. After your baby is born you get a lot of handouts, paperwork, and information from the nurses and doctors. It's really helpful to have places to store papers and write down all of the things you're told because you are definitely not going to remember everything they tell you right before you are discharged and sent home. I decided

to use my notebook to also write down questions that I might think of at home so that I wouldn't forget to ask them while at the pediatrician's office. I also used my notebook to write down when my first son ate, what side he ate on, how long he ate for, and when he had wets and dirties. I used the notebook up until he was five months old to write down his feeding schedule, otherwise I would forget when he last ate and from what side he ended on (now I just use the notepad on my phone!). It's really nice to have a special place to put all of that, and you can bring it in and show the doctor so when she asks how often baby eats, you won't be like, "Uh, a few times a day?" The folder is really handy because you get a lot of paperwork at the hospital and instead of shoving it all in your bag where it will get crumpled and ripped, you can nicely store it in your folder and keep it organized so you know exactly where it is when you get home and look for that breastfeeding handout you need. And if you decide to go to baby classes at the hospital you can also use the notebook and folder for information you get there!

23. Get a package of milk freezer bags. If you get a breast pump (which I recommend), having a box of milk storage freezer bags is really helpful. Sometimes baby decides he doesn't want to eat on one side and you get engorged and feel terrible. It is super handy to have the freezer bags so you can pump and then save the milk that you pump so that later, if you are going to be away from your baby, there is some milk for him ready in the freezer. Sometimes you'll get engorged and it hurts super bad and you'll need to pump even a little bit so that you can sleep at night. I die a little inside when I have to throw away precious breast milk I worked so hard to pump. And when I have milk freezer bags I don't have to! Plus, you don't want to send your husband on a late night or early morning run to

the store to look for them because if we're being honest, he probably won't get the right thing (Do they ever?).

24. Look up a newborn photographer and baby poses. Some hospitals have contracts with baby photographers and they will actually come to your room while you're there and take pictures. We were lucky and had the chance to get our first two babies' pictures done while we were still in the hospital. Check to see if your hospital has something like this and, if they don't, you might want to start looking around for a newborn photographer. Or, if you want to save money but still want pictures of your perfect baby, you can look online at the many tutorials on how to photograph babies on your own. I also spent a lot of time looking at baby pose ideas, and even though we had pictures taken in the hospital, I took some at home based on the pictures I saw online. If you're doing baby announcements this is especially handy because once your baby is born you don't want to have to try and look around for a photographer and ideas of how you might want to pose your baby. The last thing you want to do after giving birth is to stress about finding the perfect photographer and getting good pictures. It's nice to plan ahead and have that all set up beforehand.

25. Make Daddy feel special. I already mentioned this earlier in the book, but I made my husband a "New Dad Kit" before our first baby was born to let him know how much I appreciated him and the support he gave me (and would eventually give me during labor). I included some soap, Pop Rocks, tissues, a few books about daddies, a baby outfit with his favorite sports team's logo, Sour Patch Kids, Diet Mt. Dew, air freshener, earplugs, and a few other little personal things. Not only was it fun for me to make (and took a lot of time), it was nice to be able to

give him something special after he had given me something so special (aka his baby juice).

26. Set up baby's room. When your baby is born, you want to make sure that his nursery is ready! You don't want to come home to a room that isn't completely set up because, honestly, you are not going to want to set it up after you have just given birth. It doesn't have to be fancy, but you want it to be somewhere peaceful that you'll enjoy being. And having it all done before your baby is born is a great way to take care of that nesting instinct!

27. Pick out baby's "going home outfit." And also bring a backup! For our son, we had this super cute little outfit picked out. Unfortunately, the bottoms were way too big and we had to bring him home in a little sleeper. For our daughter, we brought a little dress and it fit great. You can't be sure how big or small your baby is going to be, so bring two outfits that will work. It's so fun picking it out while you are pregnant and imagining how your little one will look in it! And be aware of the season, too. If it's winter, you probably aren't going to want your baby to go home in short-sleeves, even if it is an adorable outfit!

28. Decide where your baby is going to sleep when she comes home. For the first few nights with our first son, he slept on our floor next to the bed in a little bassinet. We had planned that, so we had it all ready when we came home from the hospital. With our daughter, we decided to put her in her crib the first night. Our second son slept in a pack n' play at the foot of our bed for two weeks before we moved him into his room. It doesn't make a huge difference where you put your baby, but you want to be ready when you get home. Whether it's a crib, a portable bassinet, or a pack n' play, know where you are going to put your baby when you get home from the hospital, and

make sure she will be sleeping flat on her back without any loose blankets or pillows.

29. Set up a designated changing station. You want to make sure you have a place that will have wipes, diapers, and diaper cream handy. And if you're having a boy, you want to include some gauze pads and ointment for post-circumcision care. If you have a single-level home, you can just set up one spot in the baby's nursery (probably a changing table). If you have multiple levels in your house, it might be best to set up a spot on each floor. That way you won't have to always be running around when baby needs a change.

30. Buy baby Tylenol. When your baby gets his shots, you are going to feel super bad for him. He will cry and it will be so sad, and you will just want to take away his pain. Buy some baby Tylenol so that when the time comes and your baby is in pain, you will have it right there and you will have a way to help. And make sure you ask your baby's doctor before you give it to your baby. Dosage is different for little babies!

31. Register for your baby. One of the best parts of being pregnant is getting to register for your baby. I already talked about what you should put on your registry, but make sure you actually create your registry. Even if it's your second or third baby, people will still ask you what they can gift you, and it's nice to just refer them to your registry, even if all you register for are diapers and wipes!

32. Take maternity photos. Pregnancy is such a unique time in your life, and I recommend getting maternity photos taken during at least one of your pregnancies! You can even involve your husband, older siblings, or your pet!

33. Decide how you want to document your baby's growth. Something I have loved doing with all of my babies is taking monthly pictures to document their growth. And thanks to the internet, there are so many great ideas out there for ways to do it. Next to a teddy bear, on a blanket, with monthly stickers, or even in their crib. The first month goes by so fast, and you'll want to have an idea ready for how you're going to document your baby's growth!

34. Clean your car. After your baby is born, you're not going to want to (or have time to) clean your car. It's something you might not think about, but it makes a huge difference to have a clean car after your baby is born. One less thing to worry about and it definitely will give you something to do while you're waiting for baby to get here!

35. Stock up on essentials. Things like toilet paper, laundry detergent, shampoo, and conditioner are super easy to stock up on before your baby is born. If you are anything like me, you're probably going to try to avoid going to the store for the first few weeks after your baby is born (especially if it's your first!). Having essentials that you can't really live without already in your house is going to help prevent emergency trips to the store!

36. Let family members know when you want them to come. When you have a newborn, the last thing you want is a million family members coming to your house all at the same time. So, let them know when the best time to come is, especially if they live far away. For all of our kids, we had our parents come at separate times so that our house wasn't super full. And if you are totally fine with having everyone over at once, then that's awesome, too. This is your special time and you're allowed to tell people when they can and can't come over.

37. Pre-register at the hospital. Not all hospitals do this, but one of the most helpful things we did for our first two babies was to pre-register at the hospital. We sent in all of my medical information and insurance paperwork so that when it was time to go, we only had to sign a few papers before we were checked in. Call your hospital (or ask your OB) to see if you can pre-register because it really makes a difference when you check in at the hospital! Especially if you are in a hurry!

38. Have a baby shower. Having a baby shower is another super fun part of being pregnant. If nobody has offered to throw you one, ask a close friend or your mom or mother-in-law to host one for you. Especially if it's your first baby, you want to get as much help buying things as you can!

39. Buy undies you don't care about. If you haven't already heard from other moms or your doctor, your undercarriage is going to be especially tender after birth. Specifically, your lady parts are going to be especially tender after birth. You pretty much have a super heavy long period for a while, and even though the hospital gives you some disposable mesh panties, you might want to have some extra cheap ones as backup just in case. Make sure they're cotton and breathable, and definitely not too tight. You are going to be sore and uncomfortable. Get a few pairs that you won't care about if they need to be thrown away after you've recovered.

40. Buy some extra maxi pads. Going along with the last thing, you are going to be having a heavy period and won't be able to use a tampon after your baby is born. And yes, the hospital gives you some maxi pads, but you will probably go through them all and need some more once you get home from the hospital. You can even put

some in the freezer slightly damp with a mixture of water and witch hazel to help cool off your sore lady parts after delivery. So, get some maxi pads as backup and just keep them in your bathroom cabinet. It's much better to be safe than sorry in this situation! I bled for six weeks with my third and I absolutely needed more pads than what the hospital gave me!

Most importantly, just get excited! I know it's the worst waiting around for your baby. And if your due date comes and goes, you'll probably be trying to do everything you can to pass the time. Just enjoy it and try to relax. As much as you'll hate me for saying this, babies come when they are ready, not when you're ready!

Things to Do Before Your Second (Or Third, or Eighth) Baby is Born

This is an entirely separate list because when you're pregnant with subsequent babies, there are new things you'll need to do that you won't have to do with your first baby.

1. Arrange babysitting for your older child. When the time comes to go to the hospital, you need to have somewhere you can take your older child, whether it be in the middle of the night or during the day. Either have a parent come to stay, or talk to some friends or neighbors you trust who would be willing to watch your little one until you are able to go home. With my second and third pregnancies, we had a list of a few friends we trusted who were willing to watch our kids no matter when we had to head to the hospital. My mom came to stay when our daughter was born so we ended up not needing that list, but with our third baby we had some close friends watch our older two

while we were at the hospital. Either way, you need to make sure your older child(ren) will be taken care of!

2. Wash things that have been in storage for a long time. Our first child was a boy, and our second child was a girl, but there were several things that we were able to reuse that were gender neutral. White bodysuits, gender neutral-colored bodysuits, a few bibs and burp rags I sewed, some blankets, and a few of our big items that needed some spot cleaning (the car seat, bouncer, bassinet). You want to make sure that everything is clean and fresh for your new little one!

3. Get everything you need from storage. This includes things like the car seat, old clothes, jumpers, and that sort of thing. Since your kids will be at least nine months apart (probably more), I'm assuming you put things in storage. So, before your second baby is born, get those things out, assembled, and ready to go!

4. Get rid of stains. After going through several of the outfits, especially the white bodysuits from newborn days, I realized that a lot of them had stains from blowouts. I was able to get them out and have them looking nice and fresh for our second baby (you can find my tutorial for removing poopout stains on my blog)! Even though those outfits were hand-me-downs, I didn't want them to look that way!

5. Clean out the diaper bag. Having kids is messy. And every time we go somewhere, I have to make sure my diaper bag is packed with snacks. Of course, this also means that every time we go somewhere, my bag inevitably gets full of crumbs, wrappers, and other random little pieces of trash. So, if you haven't cleaned out and organized your diaper bag recently, I suggest doing it!

This may be a good time to add in a few things that you didn't have before like newborn diapers, an extra pacifier, and a nursing cover. Even if you have them in there for a few weeks before your baby is born, at least you will be ready and won't have to repack it when baby comes.

6. Pack a bag for your first child. Depending on if you're going to be taking your first child somewhere when you go to the hospital, it may be a good idea to pack a bag for them. You don't know how long your labor will last, how long your child will need to be babysat for, or if you will go into labor during the day or night. I packed little backpacks for our kids that had a pair of day clothes, a pair of pajamas, diapers/undies, wipes, snacks, and an extra sippy cup. That way, it wouldn't matter what time of day I went into labor and I wasn't worrying about grabbing everything I needed for my older kids when I was worrying about other things (like being in labor, duh). It also makes your children feel pretty special to have their own bags packed when you and baby both have bags packed.

7. Do something special with your first child. They aren't going to be an only child for much longer, so do something extra fun (like the zoo or waterpark) one last time before things change forever.

8. Make sure things work. This might result in changing batteries or even throwing things away. We quickly discovered that our original baby monitor didn't work and the batteries in our bouncer and vibrating bassinet had died. So, I called the baby monitor company and found out it was under warranty and we got it replaced (for free!), and then I replaced the batteries in the bouncer and vibrating bassinet. I also got some extra batteries to have on hand so that I wouldn't have to run to the store when

they went out in the future. You don't want to be stuck with a broken baby monitor or baby swing that won't work and no batteries when you bring your new baby home!

9. Check your insurance. Just because you had coverage or know what benefits you had with your first child, doesn't mean things are the same with your second baby. It is a good idea to make sure you know what will be covered and what you may end up paying for. Preparation is always key!

10. Make a schedule of your child's day. Obviously, everything on the schedule may not be able to be followed when you take them to a sitter or have someone come watch them, but it is nice for whoever is watching your child to know what a typical day looks like for your child. This can include things such as when your child wakes up, eats, takes naps, and goes to bed. You should also realize that there is a high possibility that this schedule will not be followed perfectly, and that's okay! At least whoever ends up watching your kids will have an idea of what your child is used to, especially regarding naptime and bedtime.

11. Write down any other helpful information for your sitter. I included extra information on the schedule I made for my son, like allergies, when he takes milk in a sippy, when he takes a pacifier, and what some of the words were that he says that we know but other people probably wouldn't figure out (like "her" for "water"). I also included my phone number and my husband's phone number because when I wrote it, I didn't know who would be watching our son and I didn't know if they would have both of our numbers. Again, it gave me peace of mind knowing that they knew how to get in touch with us should anything go wrong. And having all of this written

down before you go into labor makes it easier for you to just drop your child off and go instead of having to try and remember anything important that your sitter may need to know. Because if that's what you try to do, I guarantee you'll forget something!

12. Research double strollers. If you are having your kids close enough together that you will need to get a double stroller, it is a good idea to research which double stroller is best and which one you might want to buy. Ask friends and look on Amazon.com for reviews from other moms. The main point is to research double strollers before you just randomly pick one that is cheapest because you'll probably regret it (speaking from experience). You also may be able to find an amazing deal on your stroller if you wait a few weeks and keep checking prices. You've got a while before you have to have it, so don't impulse shop!

13. Check the expiration on your car seat. If you aren't aware, car seats expire. And if you're planning on using your first child's infant car seat for your second child, you'll definitely want to look and see when it expires. It usually says on the side or the back of the car seat when it expires, so check there first. Most car seats expire after six years, but you'll want to check your particular car seat. We were able to use our infant car seat for all three kids (because we reproduce super fast over here)!

14. Have a diaper shower. With our second baby, I was lucky enough to be able to get a lot of donated clothes from friends, I made all the burp rags I needed, and then I made a quilt and we had a few blankets already from family and friends. Everything else baby-related that we needed we decided we could just use what we had from our son. Pretty much the only thing we needed were diapers, so my good friends decided to throw me a diaper

shower! It was super helpful and I was able to get diapers that I would've had to buy for our baby anyway. A diaper shower is a great idea if you already have most of what you need, especially if your second child is going to be the same gender as your first!

Preparing for the Transition to Two Kids

Like any parent, I was excited when we found out we were expecting our second baby. But I was also worried about having two kids, especially ones only 18 months apart.

Our second baby wasn't quite as planned as our first, and I struggled more with accepting that my pregnancy was real and actually happening than the first time around.

As the months progressed and my belly grew larger, I worried about the impact a baby sister was going to have on my son. I spent all my time with him, and I was worried that when she was born, I wouldn't be able to give him enough time and attention and that I wouldn't get enough one-on-one time with him.

I also worried that I wouldn't be able to take care of my daughter like I had my son. Taking care of a newborn is exhausting, but taking care of a toddler at the same time sounded daunting. And I wanted to be able to give her the attention I gave my son, even though in my head I knew it wasn't going to be possible to sit there and hold her all the time when I also had to feed and play with my toddler.

I worried how my son was going to handle having a baby in the house. I had heard horror stories of older siblings acting out against their baby brothers or sisters, or even trying to get them sent back to the hospital. I worried that he would be jealous or regress and want to sleep in a crib or use a pacifier again when he saw his sister doing it.

I worried that I wasn't going to love my baby girl as much as I loved my son. I was worried I was going to have a favorite child or that my daughter was going to be a lot more difficult than my son and that I wouldn't connect with her as well as I did with him.

I also worried that the transition to having two was going to be harder than I thought and that I was going to become a sleep-deprived, grumpy, negative zombie that my family wouldn't want to be around.

But when we checked into the hospital knowing that we would finally meet our daughter that day, knowing that our lives were about to change forever, all of those worries seemed insignificant. I suddenly had the courage and faith that everything was going to work out. And when I held my daughter for the first time, I knew she was always supposed to be in our little family.

And when our 18-month-old son came into the room and got to hold his baby sister for the first time, my heart melted. He said "hi" to his sister and just sat there with her in his lap, staring at her. He was so gentle and sweet, and I knew I had nothing to worry about.

Yes, there were times when he wouldn't want her to touch him or he would try to play with her toys, but for the most part, he would bring her blankets and pacifiers and anything else he could find that he thought she might like. Having two kids is a million times better than having just one because you get two tiny versions of yourself, two little bodies to squeeze, four little hands to hold, and twice the love in your life.

Preparing for the transition to two kids can be intimidating and stressful and frightening, but once it actually happens, you look back on all the time you spent worrying and realize that your second baby is just as incredible as your first. And you wonder how you lived without her.

What Pregnant Women Need to Know About Postpartum Depression

Before my first son was born, I had never really heard anyone talk about postpartum depression. Even once my son was born and I filled out the new mom survey at my son's first doctor's appointment, I never really thought much about why they were giving it to me.

When my daughter was born 18 months later, I still didn't think about postpartum depression as something that was serious. Nobody talked to me about it, and I definitely wouldn't have been prepared if I had developed postpartum depression.

Now, after having three kids, I still don't see much talk about postpartum depression. It's one of those taboo but very common things women don't talk about like infertility, miscarriages, or problems breastfeeding. And even though I've never suffered from postpartum depression myself, I know a lot of people who have. And I know a lot of women who were completely unprepared for what it did to them.

Having a baby is a crazy stressful, emotional, hormonal time in your life, and sometimes it can really mess with your brain. If the feelings of anxiety and stress and sadness don't go away after two weeks[5], you may be suffering from postpartum depression. You may have heard of the "baby blues," which aren't serious and should go away after a few days or a few weeks. But if it's been two weeks and you're still depressed or have severe mood swings, cry a lot, have a hard time bonding with your baby, are withdrawing from family and friends, have a change in eating habits or sleeping habits, feel fatigued, anxious, irritable, angry, worthless, guilt, or inadequate, don't enjoy things you used to, have thoughts of harming yourself or your baby, that's not normal and you need to get help for postpartum depression.

I talked to a lot of mothers who have suffered publicly and privately, and I want to tell you a few things you should know about postpartum depression before your baby is born so you can be prepared and know how to get help if you need it.

1. Postpartum depression can happen to anyone. Having a history of mental illness in your family or yourself does not mean that you will either get it or not. Lots of women are diagnosed with postpartum depression and have no history of depression or mental disorders in their family. You might not even have postpartum depression with your first baby, but then be diagnosed with your second. Even if you don't feel depressed at all during your pregnancy, you can get it once your baby is born. There's really no way to know if you are going to have it or not, so the best way to get ahead of it is to prepare yourself before your baby is born.

2. Know that you are not alone. A LOT of women deal with postpartum depression, both silently and publicly, and having it doesn't mean that you have done something wrong or that there's something wrong with you. It's just a complication of giving birth, and up to one in seven women have it[6]. Chances are you have friends who have

postpartum depression or have suffered from it in the past. It really is nothing to be ashamed of.

3. Admitting something is wrong is the first step. If you don't feel like yourself, don't brush it under the rug. I talked to a lot of moms who had a hard time admitting that something was wrong. These symptoms are not normal, and it's 100% okay if you need help to deal with them! The first step to getting help is to admit that there is a problem.

4. Don't be afraid to ask for help. You may not be able to fight postpartum depression on your own, so once you've admitted something is wrong, ask for help. It's totally fine (actually it's great!) to ask for help. You shouldn't be shy about having postpartum depression and you don't need to hide it (that definitely won't help). Be open about what you are going through and know that it's good to talk about it.

5. Talk to someone and get the support you need. So many of my friends said that once they admitted something was wrong and talked to their doctor, things slowly started getting better. Doctors can help you by finding counseling or support groups and prescribing medication. It might take a few tries to find a doctor or therapist who listens and understands what you are going through, but don't give up. One of my friends told me that online support groups were very helpful, too. Find one where you can talk to other moms going through postpartum depression. It will help you see that you really aren't alone!

6. Medication can really help. Sometimes talking about what's going on isn't enough, and your body will need a little more to start the healing process. Antidepressants can really help you get into a different mindset and start

feeling a little better. You also might have to try different kinds before you find one that works for you, so be patient.

7. Reduce stress after the birth of your baby any way you can. Don't move two months after your baby is born, don't offer to plan a big party or school fundraiser with a newborn in the home, and don't plan on renovating your kitchen as soon as you get home from the hospital. Stress won't help, so do what you can to help reduce stress and prepare before your baby is born so you will be ready for the transition.

8. Postpartum depression can happen up to a year after your baby is born. You always need to be aware of how you are doing and take care of yourself, even after your baby is a few months old.

9. Use the Edinburgh Postnatal Depression Test. This is usually given to you at the hospital and your baby's two-week appointment, and usually again at your postpartum OB/GYN visit, but you should take it even after that just to see how you are doing. It will help you see any red flags and notice things you might not otherwise. Print it out and keep it as a resource for yourself.

10. Try to avoid any triggers that cause you stress or anxiety. If you think having meals brought to your house will stress you out because you have to answer the door, arrange for freezer meals to be brought before your baby is born. If holding your baby too much causes you stress or anxiety, ask someone else (your husband or a close friend) to hold your baby every once in a while. Breastfeeding might stress you out and make you feel depressed and, if that's the case, it might not be for you. Bottles and formula exist for a reason and you definitely

aren't a bad mom for feeding your baby formula. Just know what triggers set you off and try to avoid them.

11. Dismiss people who belittle you or make you feel bad. Unfortunately, some people don't understand or don't accept postpartum depression as a real thing. And if someone is making you feel bad because you haven't connected with your baby or you don't want to go out for a girls' night, dismiss them and move on. You don't need anyone in your life who isn't going to be on your side, and having them around will only make things worse.

12. Give your family permission to tell you if they see you exhibiting signs of postpartum depression. Sometimes you might not realize what's happening, but others close to you will. So before your baby is born, tell your husband or your mom or sister or whomever you are close to that if they notice that you're withdrawing to let you know. Like I said, you never know if you are going to suffer from postpartum depression, and telling your family what the warning signs are and having them help you just in case is a good thing.

13. Postpartum depression can happen with adoptive mothers, too. I know this book is geared toward pregnant women, but if you happen to read this and are in the process of adoption, just be aware that you could get postpartum depression, too. It never hurts to be prepared and informed.

14. If you are religious, turn to God through prayer, scripture study, church worship, and relying on Jesus. I know this tip isn't for everybody and I'm not saying that things will immediately get better, but growing closer to Christ and feeling His love for you will help.

15. It can get better. Through small steps, you can fight and overcome postpartum depression. It's not easy and it doesn't happen overnight, but there is always hope and there are always people who will support you and lift you up. Don't ever give up, and don't ever stop trying. Your baby, your family, and your friends need you.

Postpartum depression is scary, and it's something so many mothers face. But you don't have to face it alone, and knowing about it and knowing the warning signs and how to fight it before your baby is born can give you a head start if you do end up getting diagnosed with postpartum depression.

What to Pack in Your Hospital Bag

With each baby, I had my bags packed and ready to go a month before my due date. I spent hours looking at what other people recommended packing in my bag and, honestly, not a lot of it was helpful. I packed what people told me and when I got to the hospital, I didn't use half of it. There were a few things I didn't even take out of the bag! I changed a lot of things from my first to my third pregnancy, and I feel like I know pretty well what will help the most while you're at the hospital.

First, I have a big tip for you. Pack everything you can live without for a month and set that aside. Then, for things like your camera or phone charger, write those all on a little list and put them on top of your bag so that when the time comes to head out, you have a list of what you need to grab and you won't forget anything. This was awesome when the time came for us to head to the hospital because we weren't scrambling to remember what we needed to bring and it was easy to just throw it all together and head out the door. So really, pack everything you can live without for a month, and then make a little list of the other things you will need to grab before you leave.

What to pack in your hospital bag also very much depends on you. I have always worn hospital gowns and the socks they provide while I'm recovering, and I haven't ever changed into my own clothes at the hospital until it was time to go home. You might be that way too, or you might want to wear your own clothes as soon as you get into your postpartum room. You also might have no desire to shower at the hospital (me!), or you might want to get clean and wash up as soon as you can after childbirth. If you're not sure whether or not you want to bring something, bring it just to be safe. It's better to have it than not, and you don't want to make your husband run home to grab something if he doesn't have to.

Here's what to pack in your bag that you can live without for a month:

1. Travel-sized toiletries: toothpaste, shampoo, conditioner, body wash, lotion, contact solution (if needed), deodorant, chapstick, and face wash. It's nice to buy travel-sized items because they take up less space, and you can pack them before it's time to head out.

2. Flip-flops for the shower. If you're going to use the shower, bring some flip-flops. It's just like at summer camp when you had to bring flip-flops for the showers because 1,000 other people had been in there before and you didn't want to get athlete's foot.

3. Slippers. Hospital floors are cold and gross, so grab some slippers. They're nice to have when you get out of

bed to go to the bathroom or to walk around anywhere else.

4. Socks. Your hospital room might be chilly at night, or you may just have a thing about wearing socks when you are sleeping (like me). So, pack a few pairs of socks that you can wear while you are there (especially if you don't want to bring slippers).

5. Notebook and pen. The nurses and doctor tell you a lot of information before you leave the hospital. And, you also might have a lot of questions before you leave the hospital. So, it's nice to have a special place to write any information down so that you have it in one place and won't lose it when you get home.

6. Folder. You get a lot of paperwork when you have a baby, and it's really helpful to have a folder you can put it all in so you don't crush it in your bag or lose it.

7. Outfit to go home in. Obviously, you can't wear the lovely hospital gowns home, so make sure you bring an outfit for yourself to go home in. I highly recommend something loose that you wore during pregnancy. The first time I brought some pants and a shirt that I wore in the beginning of pregnancy and they were both way too tight, making me feel extra chubby and bad about myself. Sweatpants and a loose, comfortable t-shirt are great options.

8. PJs or other clothes to wear at the hospital. Like I said, you might want to just wear a new hospital gown every day, but you also might not like the way they feel. So, pack a few pairs of clothes or pajamas to wear while you're there just in case.

9. Plastic bag for laundry. When you get to the hospital, you obviously have to change into a hospital gown, and having a plastic bag to put your street clothes in is nice because then they don't get mixed up with everything else in your bag (especially if your water breaks before you get there and your clothes get all wet).

10. Nursing pads. When your milk first comes in, it is like a waterfall and it's very leaky as your body adjusts to how much your baby will drink. Bring some nursing pads so you don't leak through all your shirts.

11. Nursing bra. While it is possible to nurse your baby using regular bras, nursing bras are the best! They clip down so you can just reveal one breast at a time and that way you don't have to awkwardly move your bra around to feed your baby. Get one that doesn't have underwire to wear in the beginning.

12. Lanolin. This is probably one of the most important things! Lanolin is really helpful in the first few weeks of breastfeeding. It helps protect your nipples and heal them when they start getting chapped. I use a ton of it when I first start breastfeeding. One of the hospitals I delivered at gave me a sample and one didn't, so make sure you bring some just in case.

13. Hair ties. Should you really ever go anywhere without a hair tie? They're great at the hospital because you can pull your hair back during childbirth, you can keep it out of the way during nursing, or if you're like me and decide you don't want to shower, you can just keep it pulled back the whole time you're there.

14. Underwear you don't care about. If you follow my list of things to do before your baby is born you'll have some

on hand. Why? Because birth gets messy and you're going to bleed a lot afterwards. Yes, you will have pads down there, but if they leak, you don't want to be ruining your favorite underwear. Plus, since things get very sensitive after birth, you want to make sure you have comfy underwear that won't be suffocating your lady parts.

15. Birth plan. A birth plan is a paper that tells the nurses and doctors at the hospital what you want and don't want to do during labor and postpartum. Again, I'll talk more about it soon, but if you write one out, make sure you put it in your hospital bag!

16. Music. Labor can take a long time, and you may use music either to pass the time or to help you relax during contractions. And, make sure whatever it is you're bringing is charged and has headphones or a speaker!

17. Nursing pillow. I love these dang things. I've used the same one for all three of my babies. It helps a ton, especially in the beginning of breastfeeding when I was trying to figure out the best way to hold my son and to get comfortable myself. I have tried using just a regular rectangular pillow and it's really not the same. Get a nursing pillow and bring it to the hospital so that you can start breastfeeding off on the right foot.

18. Zip-up jacket. If your hospital room is cold, you'll want to have a jacket handy so you don't freeze. You want to try and be as comfortable as you can since you just had a baby and you deserve it!

19. Maxi pads. One of the hospitals I delivered at gave me a bunch of pads, and the other one didn't. I brought some extras all three times. Even though I didn't end up using them, it was nice to have them just in case. Every hospital

is different and you may not like the ones that you are given, or you may not be given any. And, you will want these for all that leakage your body will be doing after birth. Trust me, they are necessary.

Here's what to pack right before you leave (I recommend writing this all down on a piece of paper and putting it right on top of your packed bag):

1. Makeup. It depends on the person, but I wanted to make sure I didn't look how I felt when I was at the hospital. And, it was nice for me to be able to wash my face and do my makeup at the start of each day. It was sort of a morale booster every morning (and I also felt better about visitors coming).

2. Camera and charger. A camera is one of the most important things you can bring to the hospital. Yes, your phone takes pictures, but cameras are better. You want to document your time there so you can remember it later. We took tons of pictures at the hospital with each baby, and I love looking back at them now. And make sure you bring your charger! Also, if your memory card isn't super big, it's not a bad idea to bring a second one.

3. Phone and charger. Again, super important. I'm sure you'll want to tell all your family members who aren't there with you pretty soon after the baby is born. My phone was also a good distraction in the beginning of labor, too, because I played games on it and messed around on social media. And don't forget your charger because your phone is going to be super busy getting calls and texts of congratulations after your baby is born. And if it dies, you will be sad, and it's better not to have to send your husband home to get it for you.

4. Toothbrush. Obviously, you need to use this up until you leave the house for the hospital, and you will definitely want it while you are at the hospital. I don't think it needs much explanation.

5. Contacts or glasses. If you need them, make sure you bring them so your bundle of joy isn't a blur of joy.

6. Tablet or laptop (for entertainment in case your labor takes a long time). This isn't necessary, but it can be helpful if you want to make sure you have things to do during labor. Especially if it's your first baby and you don't know how long it will take; it's nice to have something to do while at the hospital!

7. Wallet/purse. I'm not going to explain why you need this. I think it's pretty obvious.

Like I said, it really depends on you and what you think you're going to want to bring to the hospital. And if you end up not using everything in your bag, no big deal. It's better to be prepared!

What to Pack in Your Baby's Hospital Bag

First of all, I highly recommend having separate bags. You will want to be able to find everything easily while you are at the hospital, so it just makes a lot of sense to pack things separately. Second, if this is your first baby, I recommend using your diaper bag as your baby's hospital bag. It's nice because you can get some of the stuff in there that you want to pack in a diaper bag anyway, and second, it's the perfect size. And if you're like me, you're probably eager to start using your diaper bag, so why not use it to pack your baby's things for the hospital?

One more thing. I packed a lot of things for my first baby when we went to the hospital. I used almost none of it. Yes, it's important to be prepared just in case you do need something or you decide you want to change baby into new clothes from home every day, but it's helpful to ask your hospital what kinds of things they provide. For example, diapers and wipes are things that hospitals provide, so you don't need to pack those and they are not on my list. Call ahead or ask while you're taking your hospital tour so you don't have to fill your baby's bag with unnecessary things.

And again, just like with your hospital bag, you may not use all of these things, so try and know yourself and what you're going to want to do.

1. Two or three pairs of pajamas. The button-up ones are best for newborns and little babies because when you change their diapers you don't have to take their whole outfit off. And make sure they have little feet in them to keep their toes warm!

2. Going home outfit. Our son went home in an outfit that was not his designated going home outfit, so maybe bring two outfits just in case. You don't know how big or small your baby is going to be!

3. Burp rags. Whether your baby is a spitter or not, it's nice to have some of these to burp your baby with after he eats.

4. Receiving blanket. Hospitals usually have blankets you can use, but if you have a special one you want to use, bring it!

5. No-scratch mittens. Babies are pretty much born with claws, and it's super hard to file them or clip them when they are newborns. If you have your baby wear tops that have built-in mittens then you won't really need them to wear mittens as well, but in tops without those little fold-over mittens, you want to put mittens on them. Otherwise they will scratch their little faces and you will feel absolutely terrible.

6. Pacifier. If you're planning on using one, pack one, but if you're not, don't. I didn't plan on using pacifiers for our babies until they were a few weeks old. If you are nursing your baby, you might not want to give him a pacifier for a few weeks, but if you are going to give him a bottle from the beginning, it doesn't matter.

Everyone is different with what they will use, and I really do recommend calling the hospital to see if they will have diapers and wipes and lotion for your baby. Those things take up quite a bit of space in your bag, so if you don't have to pack them, super!

What to Pack in Your Husband's Hospital Bag

I've only packed a bag for my husband once, and it was with my second baby. The first time he just went home to change and shower, and the third time he only slept at the hospital the first night and then went home to sleep with our other two kids. But having a bag for your husband is great if he is planning on staying at the hospital overnight.

Men definitely don't need as much because, first of all, they are not giving birth and, second of all, they are men. So, unless you married a high-maintenance guy, packing his hospital bag will be easy.

Basically, all he's going to need is a few changes of clothes (including underwear), socks, pajamas (if he doesn't want to sleep in his clothes), a toothbrush, and toothpaste.

Men are easy to pack for.

What to Include on Your Birth Plan

When I was pregnant with my first baby, the OB office gave me this awesome little booklet filled with information on what to expect and on the hospital I was going to deliver at. One of the most helpful things it had in it was a little birth plan for me to fill out and take to the hospital when it was time for our baby to be born. Not only was it great for me to be able to write down my preferences for our son's birth, but it helped bring me peace of mind that what I wanted for our delivery would be respected as long as it was safe for me and the baby. Even though I talked about some of these things with the doctor beforehand, it was nice to have it all written down to help my doctor remember (because doctors have a lot of patients!).

With my third baby, I wanted to put together my own birth plan and think about the things that I wanted the nurses and doctor to know when I went in. The hospital I delivered at didn't have a cool packet with a birth plan in it like the hospital my first two babies were born in, so I did a lot of research on what to include on a birth plan and came up with my own!

Before I tell you what to include, keep in mind that sometimes things don't always go as planned. Your birth plan should discuss your ideal birth situation, but you also need to remember to be flexible when the time comes and not freak out if you can't do everything the way you wanted. Sometimes you have to have a C-section instead of a vaginal birth, sometimes your baby has to be taken care of by the NICU team before you can hold him, and sometimes labor goes much quicker than you might have planned and you won't be able to get an epidural. Your birth plan is like plan A, and sometimes changes must be made for your health or the health of your baby.

The most important part of a birth plan is to consider all possible situations so you can prepare ahead of time and you won't have to make decisions when you are in the moment and your nurse is asking you what you want to do.

If you decide to print out your birth plan and bring it to the hospital, here are some things to include:

1. Names. Your name, your labor partner's name (usually your husband), your doctor's name, your doula's name (if you have one), and your baby's name (if you've decided already).

2. Due date. It will probably be on your chart, but it's nice to include it so everyone knows how far before or past your due date you are.

3. Things you would like during labor. This could include who you want with you (for me, just my husband and nobody else), if you have a playlist you want to listen to, if you want a mirror for your baby's birth (This sounds awful to me, but my sister said it really helped her push out her baby), if you'd like to have ice chips, jello, or popsicles for "nourishment" (Since that's all you can have, it's nice to make it known if you want those things), if you want to have any pictures or videos taken, if you

want constant fetal monitoring or intermittent, if you have your own delivery gown you'd like to wear, if you want to be coached during pushing or to push when you feel ready, and if you'd prefer to break your water on your own.

4. Things you would like to help relieve the pain during labor. Number one, if you want an epidural or not (in my case, **YES** in big bold letters), and if you want it offered as soon as possible or when you ask for it. Or, if you don't want an epidural, you can talk about what kinds of pain management you want to try. This part can also include if you want to use a birthing ball, to walk around, to use aromatherapy, massage, a tub (if available), if you want to stay in your bed or move around, if you prefer a certain position during birth, if you plan to use meditation or hypnobirthing methods, and if you'd like to use hot and cold packs.

5. Things you would like immediately after delivery. Things like if you want your partner to cut the umbilical cord or if you want to delay cord clamping, if you plan on doing anything with your baby's cord blood, if you want to hold the baby immediately after he is born or after he is cleaned up, if you want baby's little footprints in a special book, if you want your baby to do skin-to-skin with you or your partner, if you want to try and breastfeed immediately after delivery, if you'd like to try the breast crawl, if you'd like to have a lactation consultant come (helpful especially for first-time moms), if you'd like your baby to stay in your room as long as possible or get taken to the nursery (if your hospital has one) to be evaluated, and if you want your partner to go with your baby if they need any special care outside of the delivery room.

6. Special requests if a C-section is needed. Of course, you probably don't want this to happen, but it's good to think about it just in case. This could include seeing or holding the baby immediately after, and if you want to have the drape lowered so you can watch your baby be born.

7. Concerns and fears. This is something my first birth plan had on it and I really liked it. Especially helpful if you are a first-time mom.

8. Other things. Would you be willing to have an episiotomy, if you plan to exclusively breastfeed or not, if you plan on using a pacifier or not, if you want your baby circumcised (if he's a boy, obviously), if you tested positive for strep B (if you did, this is important to include), if you are planning on having a VBAC, and if you want to do anything with the placenta.

Every hospital is different and some won't be able to accommodate all of your requests, so be prepared for that. These are just helpful pointers on what to include on your birth plan because having a birth plan is a great way to prepare for the birth of your child emotionally as well as physically (since you can think ahead of time about different scenarios and your preferences for your child's birth). Like I said before, sometimes things don't always go as planned, and even if you had planned on doing something one way you might not be able to (like getting an epidural, breastfeeding immediately after baby is born, or even having a vaginal birth). But writing and bringing along a birth plan will definitely help everyone be on the same page when the time comes to meet your little one!

Ways to Stay Calm and Prepare for Labor and Delivery

One of the biggest things you're probably worrying about as you get closer to your due date is labor and delivery. How in the world are you supposed to prepare to push a watermelon out of a hole smaller than a golf ball?

Luckily, there are doctors, nurses, midwives, and doulas, and lots of ways to deal with pain that can help you get through it. But, despite the comforts and medical advances we have today, childbirth can still be daunting, especially when it's something you've never experienced before. It's totally normal and 100% okay to be scared (In fact, it might be odd if you weren't a little nervous!).

If we're being honest, childbirth is my favorite part of pregnancy. I know that sounds crazy, but it can really be a great experience when you go into it with positivity and excitement, knowing that you are about to meet your baby!

If you're not on the excitement train yet, that's okay. Here are some things you can do to stay calm and prepare yourself for labor and delivery:

1. Do things you can to get ready. One of the most helpful things you can do to prepare for labor and delivery is to have everything ready at home. For example, pack your hospital bag early, have baby's nursery set up, if you have family who want to visit from out of town let them know when you want them there, or do anything else off the list a few pages back. Preparing at home as much as you can is going to make it so much calmer when the time does come to leave for the hospital. You won't be rushing around trying to pack your hospital bag or stressing that

you don't have any newborn diapers yet. You'll be ready because you've prepared.

2. Don't read horror stories about childbirth gone wrong. I feel like maybe this is a "duh" thing, but I'm going to say it anyway because sometimes people don't think. Don't google stories about women who have had bad experiences with childbirth. Yes, things can go wrong, but reading about them will just freak you out and you don't need that.

3. Talk to your doctor or midwife about any concerns you have. This is a great, easy way to help you stay calm and prepare for labor and delivery. They will have solutions to probably any fear you have about childbirth. And you're presumably going to have them there during delivery, so communicating and being on the same page is very important. You'll know you're getting accurate information instead of information your mom's sister's step-daughter's grandma told her.

4. Practice breathing and meditation. Even if you aren't planning on having a natural birth, it can help. First, it can help you get through the contractions before you're given the epidural. Second, if something does happen and you aren't able to get an epidural, you'll know how to breathe through the pain and stay more calm than you would if you hadn't practiced.

5. Accept that you can't control everything. Childbirth isn't something you can guarantee is going to go perfectly. It's okay if you can't stick to everything on your birth plan, and it's okay if you have to have a C-section instead of a vaginal delivery. The most important thing is your health and the health of the baby, and you have to accept that there are things that are out of your hands that you

can't control. Just let go a little bit and put your trust in the doctors and nurses taking care of you.

Childbirth is crazy and weird, but it's also an amazing miracle. Relax and don't worry about the "what-ifs." You should be excited and feel confident in your ability to push that baby out! When the time comes, you'll have a team of people you can trust on your side, and you'll be ready to go.

How to Tell the Difference Between Braxton Hicks and Real Contractions

They say that you'll know when you're really in labor, but that definitely didn't stop me from going to the hospital for false labor twice with my first baby. Luckily, the second time I went in I was already three days past my due date and it was a slow night so the doctor induced me, but still. If you've never experienced labor before, it's hard to tell the difference between Braxton Hicks and real contractions!

Instead of just telling you that you'll know when it's real (because that's an annoying thing to say, and there's a good chance you probably won't know), I'm going to give you some helpful tips on how to know when you're really in labor and when it's just Braxton Hicks!

First of all, you may be wondering, "What are Braxton Hicks contractions?" They're basically warm-up contractions where your uterus tightens, but they don't dilate your cervix or cause you to go into labor. They aren't usually painful, but they can be uncomfortable, and I think that's where some women get confused. I mean, if you've never been in labor before, it's hard to know for sure!

Real contractions, on the other hand, do dilate your cervix and lead to labor. They might start off without much pain, but as they continue, the pain increases, too.

Here are some helpful differences so you know if you are really going into labor or just experiencing Braxton Hicks:

Braxton Hicks contractions go away if you change positions or get up and walk around. Real contractions do not.

Braxton Hicks contractions go away if you drink some water (sometimes you can experience them when you're dehydrated). Real contractions do not.

Braxton Hicks contractions may make you uncomfortable, but usually aren't painful. Real contractions will definitely make you uncomfortable and are definitely painful.

Braxton Hicks contractions do not get closer together. Real contractions get closer together the closer you get to delivery.

Braxton Hicks contractions are sporadic and do not happen at regular intervals. Real contractions are regular, come at more frequent intervals as they continue, and last longer as they continue.

Braxton Hicks contractions do not get stronger. Real contractions do.

Braxton Hicks contractions are felt in the front of your abdomen. Real contractions are felt in your abdomen and possibly your back.

One thing that the nurses told me the first time I came in with false labor was that if you can talk through the contractions, they are probably not the real thing. That didn't really make sense to me until I actually was having real contractions. Real contractions really do hurt and you have to stop and breathe through them.

Another difference I noticed that might be helpful to note is that I actually had to feel my belly with my hands to see if it was tight to know if I was having a Braxton Hicks contraction. With real contractions, I knew without having to feel if my belly was tight and contracting, partly because of the more intense pain, and partly because I could feel it way stronger.

It was a big bummer going to the hospital twice only to have them tell me that I wasn't in labor, but at least the second time it worked out and I was able to get induced. With my third baby, I absolutely knew I was in labor, and by the time I got to the hospital, I had to stop walking and breathe through the contractions when they hit.

If you really aren't sure, it never hurts to call your doctor or to go to the hospital just in case. It might be a disappointment when they monitor you for a while and send you home, but wouldn't you rather have that happen than not getting to the hospital in time (no having babies on the side of the road, please)?

Prodromal Labor

The only thing worse than Braxton Hicks is prodromal labor.

I didn't know what prodromal labor was until I was 38 weeks pregnant with my third baby and I woke up in the

154

middle of the night with contractions that I knew were different than Braxton Hicks because they were painful and getting closer together. I timed them for a few hours, and they were getting closer together, but then all of a sudden they went away. Two nights later it happened again. And then the night after that it happened again. It sucked.

Prodromal labor is often called "false labor" and is basically when you have contractions that don't result in the birth of your baby[7]. It sucks because it feels like labor and the contractions don't go away when you get up and walk around or drink water (like Braxton Hicks), but then they just stop and you'll be left wondering what the heck just happened.

They often happen at the same time every day, and that can often be at night (like with me!). It really is the worst, and if you get them, you might feel discouraged and frustrated, especially because you're probably already hyper-aware of everything going on with your body as you not-so-patiently await labor.

If you get them, I'm sorry, and I've totally been there. Hopefully, they progress and turn into real labor soon!

Ways to Induce Labor

With each of my babies, I have gone crazy trying to get labor going. At 39 weeks, babies are considered "full term,"[8] and when you're at that point, you're probably willing to try every safe thing possible to induce labor. With each of my babies I've tried a lot of things, and while some of them are old wives' tales and I don't think many of them worked for me, they are fun to try, and they definitely keep you busy! Here are some safe things you can try to kick your baby out of his cozy home:

1. Pressure points. There are a few places on your body that if you press and rub them they can help stimulate contractions. One is between your index finger and thumb, and one is on the inside of your leg about two inches above your ankle. My husband actually talked about these in medical school, so there's some truth to them. And, if you're just sitting around watching a movie or watching TV anyway, why not make your man rub your ankle or hand? It feels good and if it works, then it's worth it!

2. Eat spicy food. Spicy food can irritate your bowels, and it can sometimes help trigger uterine contractions, making you go into labor. Unfortunately, if it doesn't work, you might spend a night pooping your guts out, but if it does, you might end up having your baby! The pros outweigh the cons in this situation!

3. Red raspberry leaf tea. Okay, so this one doesn't necessarily help induce labor, but it is supposed to help strengthen your uterine muscles and make labor shorter. I actually really do like this one and think it makes a difference. You can take it in a pill or as tea, and you can start as early as 32 weeks pregnant. I'm definitely a big proponent of this one!

4. Walk. And walk and walk and walk. Why? Walking can help your little one drop into your pelvis and put pressure on your cervix, preparing your body to go into labor. It might hurt (especially if it's your second or third pregnancy), but it can help naturally induce labor.

5. Baths. A nice, relaxing hot bath can help loosen your muscles and calm you down, making you more likely to

go into labor soon. I would recommend adding bubbles and just soaking. It helps your sore body and gives you another excuse to just lay down and relax.

6. Eat fresh pineapple. Pineapple contains an enzyme that is supposed to help soften your cervix and bring on labor. It doesn't contain much of the enzyme, so you would have to eat a ton of pineapple for it to really have a strong effect, but that will probably also make you more miserable than anything. And, it has to be fresh pineapple, too. Canning destroys the enzyme, so you want to make sure it's freshly cut!

7. Sex. No, don't say gross. This is actually true. Sperm can help thin and dilate the cervix, which is what you want when you are about to have a baby. Sex can also help trigger contractions. So, even though you may feel like a whale barely able to move, just try it. You never know!

8. Bumpy car rides or bouncing on a birth ball. With my third baby I bounced on a birth ball for three days, took a day off, and then went into labor on the fifth day. It works!

9. Walk in place and read *The Hunger Games*. Just kidding! But for real, this is what I was doing when my husband and I decided it was time to go to the hospital with our first baby!

Now, obviously, I am not a doctor and these are just things I did to try to induce labor. If they don't work, don't blame me! But at least you stayed busy, am I right?

Getting Sent Home From the Hospital

I've only been sent home from the hospital once, but it absolutely sucked. We had packed our bags, been monitoring my contractions (which turned out to be Braxton Hicks), and I'd even been walking around our little apartment to see if they'd go away. When they didn't, we decided it might be go time and got in the car for the 30-minute drive to the hospital.

When we got there and found out I wasn't dilated past a one, we were a little bummed, but we didn't know any better so we stayed hopeful. We were put in a room and I got changed into a hospital gown. The nurses started monitoring my contractions, and I loved seeing how the chart displayed each one. I thought it might actually be happening and my husband and I were so excited!

But after a few hours, the contractions started to fizzle out. Honestly, I should have known that nothing was happening because they weren't hurting at all and I had to look at the monitor to even know when they were happening. So, I changed back into my clothes and we went home with our spirits crushed.

Getting sent home from the hospital is seriously the worst. But it happens a lot to first-time mamas and even second-time mamas. The nurses won't laugh at you, and even though you'll feel pretty crappy and just want to eat ice cream the whole rest of the day (you're allowed to), you can rest assured that your baby's not going to be in your belly forever. Sometimes you'll be back within a few hours or a few days, and sometimes it might be a week or two before you're back. But you'll be back, and you'll get to meet your baby soon!

The Waiting Game

The last few weeks of pregnancy are my least favorite. They are so far from my favorite part of pregnancy that I shouldn't even include the word favorite in that sentence. The last few weeks of pregnancy are my least. That's better.

Not only are you super uncomfortable, but you're tired, too. You're excited to meet your baby, but mad that he's not here yet, and you probably hate everything.

The last few weeks of pregnancy you play the waiting game. You Google every little thing related to labor, you are extra sensitive to any movements your baby makes (Did he just drop?) and anything that sneaks out of your body (Was that my mucous plug?). You obsess and daydream about having your baby and you get addicted to reading birth stories.

If anyone dares to text or call and ask you if you've had your baby yet, you make a mental note to punch them in the face next time you see them. Don't they know that you'd announce it the moment it happens?

The end of the third trimester sucks, but the redeeming quality about it is that it really is the end. You're so close to being done with pregnancy and starting this new chapter in your life. You are a few weeks (or days) away from holding your very own baby in your arms, a baby you grew and nourished inside of you for nine months, a baby that is half you and half your husband, and is more beautiful, special, and incredible than any other baby that has ever lived.

1. Hildreth, Kerry L., et al. "Oxidative stress contributes to large elastic arterial stiffening across the stages of the menopausal transition." *Menopause*, vol. 21, no. 6, 2014, pp. 624–632., doi:10.1097/gme.0000000000000116.
2. "Pregnancy Weight Gain - Weight Gain During Pregnancy." *American Pregnancy Association*, 12 Dec. 2015, americanpregnancy.org/pregnancy-health/pregnancy-weight-gain/.
3. "Pregnancy Dreams." *American Pregnancy Association*, americanpregnancy.org/your-pregnancy/pregnancy-dreams/ .
4. "Caffeine Intake During Pregnancy." *American Pregnancy Association*, 2 Sept. 2016, americanpregnancy.org/pregnancy-health/caffeine-during-pregnancy/.
5. "Postpartum depression." *Mayo Clinic*, Mayo Foundation for Medical Education and Research, 11 Aug. 2015, www.mayoclinic.org/diseases-conditions/postpartum-depression/basics/definition/con-20029130.
6. "Postpartum Depression." *American Psychological Association*, www.apa.org/pi/women/resources/reports/postpartum-depression.aspx.
7. Murphy, Carrie. "A Quick Guide to Prodromal Labor Contractions." *Fit Pregnancy and Baby*, 3 Apr. 2017, www.fitpregnancy.com/pregnancy/labor-delivery/quick-guide-prodromal-labor-contractions.
8. "What is full term?" *March of Dimes*, Oct. 2013, www.marchofdimes.org/pregnancy/what-is-full-term.aspx.

Labor and Delivery

The Finish Line

By the end of the third trimester, you just want pregnancy to end. You are tired of being pregnant and you're excited to finally meet and hold your baby in your arms. You also might be a little bit scared about the transition you're about to go through. It's one thing in life that is truly "life-changing."

A lot of women are nervous about the actual childbirth part of pregnancy, and that's totally normal. Like I said before, it's insane that you're supposed to push a watermelon out of something the size of a golf ball. I mean, that shouldn't even be possible, right?

But seriously, I think childbirth might be my favorite part of pregnancy! Not just because it's the end and it means I don't have to be pregnant anymore, but because everything the last nine months has led to this point. It's the finish line in a nine-month marathon, and you just have to suck it up (or push it out) and reach the end. It's not going to be easy and you're going to be sore after, but the prize for finishing is absolutely worth all that hard work.

Home Births

Before I had my first baby, I don't think I even knew that people had babies at home. I had no idea what a home birth entailed and, honestly, if someone had told me her baby was born at home, I would've been like, "Did you not make it to the hospital?"

Today, lots of mamas choose to have their baby at home, and that's great! I love reading stories about home births and how mamas labor at home and give birth in their bedrooms or living rooms with the help of a midwife and their husband by their side. Where you have your baby is up to you, and you should never feel like you have to explain yourself to anyone (whether it's at home, at a birthing center, or at the hospital).

All three of my babies have been born at the hospital, and since that's what I know, I'm going to focus more on hospital births in this section. But, even if you plan on having a home birth, there's a lot of helpful information here about what to expect during delivery!

I just wanted to take a few minutes and acknowledge that some mamas have their babies at home and some choose to have their babies at the hospital. Either one is great, and we should support each other in our decisions, even if they are different from our own. We don't need any more judgment and hate in this world.

Should I Go Natural?

I think that women who decide to go natural and not have any type of pain medication are rock stars.

There are lots of different pain management techniques that don't use any type of medicine and that work wonderfully. Some focus on breathing, massage, and position changes, some focus on self-hypnosis techniques, some use water, birth balls, or squatting to help ease pain, and some focus more on creating a soothing, calm environment to help you relax and get through contractions.

There are also many benefits to going natural. Pain medications might make you completely numb and make it harder to know when to push, or they might make you a little loopy or even nauseous. You also might recover quicker from birth without any medicine in your system. You're fully connected to the experience, and labor is often shorter without any pain medication. For thousands of years, women have been "going natural." It's what our bodies were made for.

That being said, I have had epidurals for all three of my babies, and I do not regret it in the slightest. If I ever have another baby, I'll probably get another epidural. I am all about that anesthesia, baby.

Deciding to go natural or to get pain medicine is totally up to you. It's not up to your mom who went natural, your best friend who had an epidural, or even your doctor who laughs when you say you don't want any medicine (which, if that happens, get a new doctor because you want them to be on your side).

Make your decision based on how you feel. And remember that if things change, that's okay, too. You might plan on getting an epidural and not have time to, or you might plan on going natural and end up having a long labor and deciding you want some pain medicine. No matter what happens, it's okay. The most important thing is a healthy baby and a healthy mama.

Also, regardless of what you decide, I recommend at least learning a little bit about natural pain management methods. My best friend had an epidural, but her son was born so quickly the medication didn't have time to work. She basically delivered a 9lb 8oz baby boy without an epidural, and she is forever amazing in my eyes (for that and like 1,000 other reasons). So please, at least do a little bit of research on natural pain relief!

Childbirth Terms You Should Know

During pregnancy, you hear a lot of new words: amniotic fluid, placenta, gestational diabetes, fundal height. It can be a lot to take in, especially as a first-time mom! But knowing what your healthcare provider is talking about is important, especially when it comes to childbirth terms. When you know what's going on and what options you have, you're more empowered and you can make informed decisions for yourself and your baby.

Since childbirth is always different and your experiences might be different with each baby, doing a little research before you go into labor can be really helpful! Here are some childbirth terms you should know regardless of what type of birth you are planning on:

Vaginal birth. I'm assuming you know this one because duh, everyone probably does, but we're starting off with the most basic. Vaginal births are the most common type of birth, and obviously it's when your baby is born via your vagina.

Cesarean section. You probably know this one, too, and it's more commonly referred to as a C-section. A cesarean section is the delivery of your baby through an incision in your abdomen and uterus. There are a variety of reasons why this might happen. Sometimes it's planned and sometimes it's not. Either way, it's also quite common and totally fine if it happens.

VBAC. Vaginal birth after cesarean. Just because you have one C-section doesn't mean every birth you have has to be a C-section. You may be able to have a vaginal birth after!

Natural birth. This refers to going through labor and delivery without medications or interventions.

Nonstress test. A test done during pregnancy to check on baby's heart rate and movements.

Preeclampsia. A pregnancy complication characterized by high-blood pressure, swelling of the hands and feet, and protein in your urine. It's manageable, but it can also be dangerous to you and your baby (especially at the end of pregnancy).

Posterior position. When your baby is posterior, it means he is head down, but facing your abdomen (face-up).

Anterior position. When your baby is anterior, it means they are head down, but facing your back. This is the best position for childbirth.

Transverse position. When your baby is transverse, it means your baby is sideways.

Breech presentation. This means your baby is bum-down. It's not a preferred position for delivery.

Dilation. Dilation refers to when your cervix starts opening for childbirth, and it's a sign that you are progressing! You have to dilate to 10 cm to deliver your baby (sounds insane, right?).

Effacement. Effacement is when your cervix starts getting ready for delivery by thinning. As your baby engages, he will drop closer to the cervix, and your cervix starts to soften and get thinner. Your doctor or midwife will say things like "50% effaced" or "ripening." When it's 100%, that means it's go-time!

Lightening. Not to be confused with lightning, because that has nothing to do with childbirth. Lightening is when your uterus starts to drop and the head of your baby begins to engage in the pelvis. When people say your baby "drops," this is what they are talking about.

Engagement. When your baby's head enters the pelvis.[1]

Posterior placenta. When the placenta develops in the back of the uterus (along the mother's back).

Anterior placenta. When the placenta develops in the front of the uterus (along the mother's abdomen).

Placental abruption. The separation of the placenta from the uterine lining. This is bad because it can deprive your baby of oxygen and nutrients, and it generally results in pain and bleeding.

Placenta previa. When the placenta lies low in the uterus and either partially or completely covers the cervix. Later in pregnancy it can cause bleeding and other complications, and it usually requires a C-section.[2]

Rupture of membranes. Aka, when your water breaks (because they have to go and make it medical on you).

Meconium. When there is meconium in your fluid, it means your baby has pooped in utero and the NICU team will probably have to be there for the delivery to make sure your baby hasn't aspirated any feces. My first baby had this and he was totally fine.

Bradley Method. A couple-focused, natural childbirth method.

Induction. Using medication or other techniques to start labor.

Catheter. A tube that is inserted somewhere into your body to either deliver medication or drain fluid. In labor, if you get an epidural, you'll get a catheter in your bladder to drain your urine.

Early labor. The onset of labor until you are 3 cm dilated.

Active labor. Labor from 3 cm dilated to 7 cm dilated.

Transition. Labor from 7 cm to full 10 cm dilated.

Bear down. Reference to the strong urge a woman feels to push (kind of like a feeling she needs to poop) at the end of labor.

Vocalize. When you moan or groan during labor. A great way to release stress and tension and get through contractions.

Perineum. The area between your vagina and Uranus. I mean, your anus (Did you giggle?).

Episiotomy. A small incision in the perineum to prevent it from tearing during childbirth.

Cephalopelvic disproportion (CPD). When a baby's head is too big to fit through the mother's pelvis. It is one of the most common reasons to have a C-section.[3]

Dystocia. Slow or difficult labor or birth.

Shoulder dystocia. When the baby's shoulders get stuck in the birth canal after delivery of the head.

Prolapsed cord. When baby's umbilical cord falls out of the cervix before the baby does.

Vernix. A thick, cheesy-like substance that covers baby's skin in utero; sometimes it's still present at birth.

Breast crawl. The instinct of babies to find their mother's nipple and start breastfeeding. Immediately after birth, the baby is placed on his mother's chest and allowed to move towards the nipple and latch on by himself.

Skin-to-skin. When your baby is placed on your chest immediately after birth (your skin on his skin). Dads can also participate in skin-to-skin by removing their shirts and holding baby. It can be done after birth as well.

APGAR. A method used to test the health of a newborn. It's done at one minute and five minutes after birth.

I told you there were a lot of new childbirth terms you should know! It's helpful to know these terms because you never know what's going to happen, and you want to know the words that are being thrown around so you can make the best choice for you and your baby!

A Quick Note: Take Note

If you're planning on writing down your baby's birth story, take notes. Write down when you start feeling contractions, your emotions, your nurses' names, when you get checked and how far along you are, and anything else you can think of. Labor goes by so fast, and even though the birth of your child is something you'll never forget, it helps to take notes on the little details that you might not remember.

Stand Up For Yourself

I love listening to pregnancy and birth podcasts and reading birth stories, and one thing that I have heard several times is that moms wish they had stood up for themselves more during labor. You might have an amazing doctor and amazing nurses who take great care of you and listen to your requests, but you also might end up with the doctor on call whom you have never met and who just wants to make it home before dinner. There are good and bad doctors and nurses, just like in every profession.

If you feel like you aren't being treated well, stand up for yourself. If your nurse is mega grumpy and rude to you, it's okay to ask for a different one. You want your baby's birth to be a good experience, not one that you look back on and have regrets about!

Get Out!

When you're close to, at, or past your due date, you may opt for an induction. It's basically when you kick your baby out of your uterus. Sometimes it's medically necessary, sometimes it's for convenience, and sometimes it's for another reason.

I was induced with my first and second babies, and both experiences were good for me. Inductions can make contractions more painful (which happened with my first baby) and slow down labor (which happened with my second baby).

It's super hard to wait until you go into labor naturally, especially if your doctor is willing to induce you, but having been induced and having gone into labor on my own, I do recommend waiting until your body goes into labor on its own. It's better for you and your baby, and it's kind of exciting! I loved feeling the contractions getting closer together and more intense (call me crazy, but it's true). I loved knowing that my body was doing its part to go into labor and get that baby out of me (especially because I was READY).

However, sometimes you have to get induced for medical reasons, and that's totally fine. Sometimes your body won't go into labor on its own, and that's totally fine, too. It doesn't mean that something is wrong with you, and we're lucky we live in a time where we can get induced if need be.

The Beginning of the End

If you thought your body had gone through some weird stuff during pregnancy, just wait. Childbirth is a whole new ball game. Before you start labor, there are a few things your body's going to do to prepare, and it's about to get messy.

The mucus plug. Before you go into labor, you lose your mucus plug. It's basically like a giant booger in your underpants, and it's gross. It's a blob of mucus that has been in your cervix to block bacteria from getting in. It's not a great sign that labor is starting because it can "grow back" (gross, right?), and you may lose it two or three times. But it is a sign that you're getting close!

The bloody show. The mucus plug is NOT to be confused with the bloody show. THEY ARE DIFFERENT! The bloody show is a better sign that labor is coming because it means that your cervix is "ripening," getting ready for childbirth. As you begin to dilate, capillaries in your cervix begin to break, which leads to a little bit of blood in your underpants. You shouldn't have a ton of blood, it can be pink, red, or brown, you might miss it if you go to the bathroom at night, and it usually happens after you lose your mucus plug.

Diarrhea. It's gross, but as your body gets ready for labor, you may get diarrhea, or at least runny poops. As your uterus starts contracting (even if you can't feel it yet), it irritates your bowel, which makes you poop a lot. Get ready because you're probably going to get to know your toilet a little better than you would like.

171

Water breaking. Your water doesn't always break on its own, and even though it doesn't always break at the start of labor, I'm including it here. I know in movies and on TV they always show pregnant women out in public and all of a sudden their water breaks and completely gushes all over and they're like "Time to go to the hospital!" all happy and cheery. Nope. That's a pretty rare occurrence. And when it does break, it is WEIRD. It feels like you're just peeing a ton and it's all warm and weird, and with each contraction a little more comes out. It's like you're peeing more than you have ever peed before. And if there's meconium in your fluid, the NICU team will probably have to be there at the delivery to make sure your baby is okay after they're born.

So far you've got mucus, blood, poop, and amniotic fluid south of the border. And that's just the beginning, mamas!

What to Expect During Labor and Delivery

Checking in. Depending on the hospital you go to, you might have to go to a triage before getting admitted. At the hospital I went to with my first two babies, I was immediately put into a private room where I was monitored and where I stayed until delivery, but at the hospital I went to with my third baby, I had to go into a triage and get checked there before I was admitted. They were slow and took their sweet time, and I had to be 5 cm dilated before they admitted me. It was a bummer.

Getting checked. Several times throughout labor you'll have to "get checked." It's the same thing as at your OB appointments toward the end of pregnancy where they have you lie down with your knees bent and lying out to the side and they check to see how far dilated and effaced you are. It's uncomfortable. And it's even worse when you're in labor. Just be ready for it.

Monitoring. The way they monitor your baby and your contractions during labor at the hospital is with two big circle things (not the technical term) strapped to your belly. They move around a lot and, in my experience, have to be adjusted pretty often. They make it hard to get comfortable, and you obviously can't get out of bed when they're on. You can ask to be monitored intermittently, which is what I did with my third labor so I could walk around and help things progress. I just came back to the room every 30 or 45 minutes and they put the monitors on and made sure everything was still good. I much preferred this, but everyone is different!

Labor takes a long time. I guess in some situations it can go pretty fast, but in most cases (and especially for first-time moms), it takes a long time. There's a lot of waiting during labor, and it can be mega boring. Make sure you have something to do like reading a book, playing a game on your phone, or watching a movie on your laptop. It can help pass the time, and it helps when you're trying to relax so your body will do its part. My husband and I watched a lot of TV during my first and second labors.

Throwing up. You might throw up during labor. Sometimes it's because of the pain, and sometimes it's because of medication. But just be warned that it can happen (as if you need another thing to deal with besides the pain of contractions).

You can't eat during labor. Both of the hospitals that my babies were born at didn't allow women to eat during labor, just in case I had to have a C-section. The only thing they allowed was clear liquids (Sprite, water) and ice chips. I have heard that some hospitals don't even allow that. And since labor takes a long time, you should probably grab a bite to eat before heading to the hospital, and prepare to be starving after your baby is born. Also, make sure your husband knows what you want to eat after your baby is born because once you actually have your baby, you're going to want it ASAP.

Your nurse. She'll be in and out of your room while you're in labor. You'll probably get a little button you can push to request her to come in. Nurses also change every 12 hours (in my experience), so you might not have the same nurse at delivery as you do when you get checked in, which is a bummer if you really grow to like the nurse you have and then she has to leave when you're at 9 cm.

The epidural. It is dang hard to sit still for that epidural. You can't get it until you are dilated past a certain point because it can slow labor down, and usually when you are that far along it's already pretty painful. And then the anesthesiologist comes in and is like "Sit on the edge of the bed and curl your back and don't move" and you're like "Are you kidding me?" You have to sit there for a while and you'll probably have a few contractions during the process, and it's hard to sit still. It's a little scary, but once you have it in and the medicine is going, it's magic. You should also know that if you do get an epidural, you have to get a catheter (basically a tube that continuously drains your bladder) and that feels really uncomfortable when it goes in. Once you do get the epidural, you will probably have to switch sides and move positions a few times in order for it to balance out and spread evenly on both sides of your body. You'll need help to do this because your epidural will pretty much make it impossible to move from the waist down, especially at first. You might also experience shaking and chills when you get an epidural, too. My doctor husband told me that it's because the epidural medicine is cold, so when it goes in your body it feels cold and makes you feel cold. One of my mama friends also told me that you can ask for a partial epidural instead of the full dosage, which if you want to be able to feel a little bit, might be a good option for you! I'm a big fan of epidurals, but if you don't want one, that's cool, too, and we can still be friends!

You might poop. I know. This is the one you're most worried about, right? Pooping during labor sounds absolutely horrible and so incredibly embarrassing, but it's actually quite common. I wasn't able to find a statistic on it, but it happens all the time. Your doctor will have seen it, your nurses will have seen it, and it's really not a big deal. I made my husband promise me that he would never tell me if I pooped during labor, and to this day I have no idea. Because your contractions stimulate your bowels, and you use the same muscles to poop as you do to push your baby out, it might happen. And it's not a big deal.

There will be lots of people in the room. One thing that completely caught me off guard with my first baby's delivery was how many people were in the room when it was go time. Besides the nurse (probably more than one) and the doctor, there were also medical students, nursing students, and the NICU team. Plus, my husband was there. If you have any other family that you want there, they'll be there, too. It can get crowded real quick. And, yes, you're allowed to request no students be in the room if you really care (but speaking as the wife of a doctor, that's how they learn!).

By the end of labor, you have zero modesty. With everything that goes on (lifting up your gown to fix the monitors, lifting up your gown to get checked, pushing your baby out of your lady parts, trying to breastfeed after your baby is handed to you) during labor and childbirth, you'll have zero modesty by the end of it. You're basically naked when everything is over. You probably won't care about nursing your baby with the nurses and doctors in the room, and you certainly will be used to having people inspect your lady parts. I'm a pretty modest person (I don't even like nursing in public with a cover), but during childbirth that's all thrown out the window. And it's not like you're the first naked woman in labor your nurses and doctors have seen, so don't worry about it.

Pushing. Don't expect to push through two or three contractions and suddenly have your baby. Most women have to push for a long time before their babies are born. Don't push until your body is ready (you'll feel like you need to poop because of the pressure of your baby's head). The best advice I can give you is to push like you're trying to poop. Yes, you might poop, but like I said, it's not a big deal and that's common. I have pushed out three babies and every time I've pushed using my lower ab muscles like I'm pooping and it has worked great for me.

The ring of fire. Ever hear someone talk about the ring of fire? The ring of fire is when your muscles and skin around your lady parts are stretching as far as they can as your baby's head comes out. It's also called crowning. I haven't felt it since I've had epidurals all three times, but I've heard it's incredibly painful and that even with an epidural you can still feel it sometimes.

What to Expect After Your Baby is Born

Congratulations! You are now the mother of a beautiful newborn! But the hard part isn't over yet. Your body still has a few more things to deal with that you should be aware of.

Delivering the placenta. It might seem super obvious to some people, but I completely forgot about delivering the placenta when my first baby was born. After your baby is born, you have to push again and deliver the placenta. It might be easy; it might be hard. After my first baby it was easy, but after my second baby, the placenta broke inside of my uterus and the doctor had to scrape it out and push on my stomach to help free it up. That was very painful, even with the epidural I'd had. Hopefully, it's easy for you, but just know that you still have a little work to do after your baby comes out.

Stitches. If you tear at all (I have with all three babies and it's super common), you'll probably have to get a few stitches. The doctor will do it right after your baby and placenta are delivered, and the most I've ever felt is a little tugging while they did it. Depending on if you get an epidural or not, you might feel more or less. You can get local anesthetic for this, too.

Meeting your baby. Let your doctor and nurse know if you want to immediately hold your baby and delay weighing and cleaning. If your baby is healthy and there aren't any concerns, they should let you do skin-to-skin immediately. I wasn't able to do this with my first baby because there was meconium in my amniotic fluid and they had to make sure he hadn't ingested it, but I did with my second and third babies and it was magic. So, let them know what you want to do, and don't be too upset if you can't. Remember, a healthy baby is the most important thing.

Going to the bathroom the first time. When you're all done and ready to change and get cleaned up, your sweet, sweet nurse will help you into the bathroom and she will show you how to take care of yourself postpartum. She'll help you get some of those nice mesh cotton undies on and help you get the big maxi pads in there. She'll show you how to gently rinse off with a squirt bottle after you go to the bathroom and how to use dermoplast spray to help ease the pain. Don't be shy (like you would be after all you've been through) and let her help you. You might feel super awkward, but you need her help, and after you'll feel so grateful!

Peeing after the catheter. If you got an epidural and had to have a catheter, be warned that peeing after it comes out is a little hard at first.

Postpartum pooping. It's also hard to poop postpartum. Make sure you take those laxatives they give you, eat lots of fiber, drink lots of water, and just relax. Try not to push very much and just let it happen.

Postpartum bleeding. You're basically going to have a heavy period for a week or two, and then lighter bleeding for 2-4 more weeks. Your doctor will tell you 4-6 weeks, but my last one was closer to 7 weeks before I stopped bleeding. DO NOT use a tampon, and just change those maxi pads often. They get smelly and it's gross, but it will end, I promise.

Squishy stomach. Another thing I probably should've realized after my first baby was born but didn't was the Jell-O belly. This is what I call how squishy and weird your stomach is after your baby is born. Obviously you're not going to go back to normal immediately, but it really caught me off guard the first time!

You may not want to shower or get dressed in the hospital. I brought my own clothes and shower stuff to the hospital with all three of my children's births, but I did not use them once. And that's totally okay if that's you. You may just want to stay in hospital gowns the whole time you're there and wait to shower until you get home. You also might want to wear your own clothes. Either way, it's okay. Don't feel a ton of pressure to look your best. You just had a baby, and you're amazing!

Sore boobs. Whether or not you choose to breastfeed, your breasts are going to hurt for a few days as your supply either adjusts or dries up. One of my mama friends told me that putting clean cabbage on your boobs can really help ease the pain of engorgement! And use lots of lanolin if you're breastfeeding because it will protect your poor little nipples.

Having a baby is absolutely crazy. Our bodies are amazing and it's wild that they can grow a human baby and then push it out and we can get up and walk around so soon after. Don't be too hard on yourself if it takes a while to recover. You're a boss, no matter what kind of birth you have.

When Things Don't Go According to Plan

You can plan all you want for the perfect birth, but things don't always go according to plan. Remember that birth plan we talked about? Don't get too attached because you might have to throw it out the window (figuratively, of course, please don't litter).

Yes, it's important to prepare as much as you can and know what kind of childbirth experience you would like, but you can't always predict what's going to happen, especially during childbirth. The number one most important thing during childbirth is a healthy baby and a healthy mom. That might mean that you have to get an emergency C-section, or that even though you wanted to go natural you end up getting induced and getting an epidural. That's totally okay. *There's no wrong way to have a baby* (whether that's in the hospital with an epidural or at home in the water with a midwife). Mentally prepare yourself for things not going according to plan by trying to stay positive and keeping baby's health as your top priority.

I've heard women talk about having traumatic childbirth experiences, or not having the peaceful, natural births they had planned for. It's hard when birth doesn't go the way you want. It's hard when you've prepared for something for nine months (or longer if you wanted a certain kind of childbirth long before pregnancy) and then it doesn't happen. It's okay to grieve for a little bit, too. But that's part of childbirth. Try to find a way to make peace with the birth that you have. There's no use stressing about something in the past that you can't change!

March 6, 2013 – The Birth Story of Jameson Daniel Johnson

By the end of pregnancy, I was so ready to meet my baby (Doesn't every birth story begin like that?). My husband and I were doing everything we could to try to induce labor naturally. We spent almost every night walking around the mall, and I was eating lots and lots of spicy food (and antacids).

The night I was 39 weeks, I could feel myself having contractions. They didn't hurt at all, but I could tell my belly was tightening and they were a little more than five minutes apart (little did I know these were Braxton Hicks). We went to bed and when I woke up, I was still having them, and they were a little closer together. We grabbed all of our bags and headed to the hospital.

I was checked in and we were told that while I was having contractions, I was still 1 cm dilated (which I had been at every OB appointment). After three hours, the contractions started to go away and they sent us home telling me that when they started to hurt and I couldn't talk or walk through them to come back.

The next few days were pretty hard because I had gotten so excited that he was going to come a bit early, and then we had been sent home. I was uncomfortable, grumpy, and just wanted to hold my baby in my arms. I kept doing things that week to try to induce labor, but nothing was working. I would have contractions on and off, but they never got strong and they always went away.

My due date came and went. I had been taking weekly pictures, but I was so grumpy about still being pregnant that I didn't take an "official" bump picture. Then Sunday came and went, then Monday, and then we got to Tuesday. I was 40 weeks and three days and, throughout the day, my contractions started getting a little more intense. They weren't going away, and by 3:30 p.m. I decided I was probably in early labor. I was having a hard time breathing through the contractions (or I was making myself think I was), and while I was hopeful, I tried not to be too optimistic because I didn't want to go to the hospital and get sent home again.

That night I made dinner and was trying to do things to distract myself while still trying to get labor going. I was walking in place while reading *The Hunger Games*, and the contractions were progressively getting a little stronger. At this point, I wasn't really timing them because I didn't think they were strong enough, and it kept getting me down because they hadn't been consistent. Around 7:30 p.m., I went to the bathroom and noticed some blood. I got excited, but it wasn't that much, so I told my husband that if there was a little more we would call the doctor. Around 8 p.m., I went to the bathroom again and noticed quite a bit more blood, so we called the doctor and she told us to come on in and get checked out. Once again, we loaded our bags in the car and left for the hospital.

We got checked in at 8:30 p.m. and found out I hadn't progressed and was still only 1 cm dilated. Needless to say, I was pretty frustrated. When my doctor came in, we told her that we had an appointment the next day to get a nonstress test and an ultrasound, and she said that since it was a slow night on the labor and delivery floor, and because we'd probably schedule an induction soon anyway, she would just go ahead and induce me that night. Honestly, I would've hugged her if I hadn't been on the bed with the belly monitors strapped to me! We said thank you like a million times, and she said to start me on Pitocin around 11:30 p.m.

I was still having some contractions on my own, and they were getting closer, so we walked around and I drank some liquids to get things moving. Walking helped my contractions get stronger, and after a while I was having to stop because they were hurting. Looking back now, I'm 100% sure I had no idea what it meant to have a contraction truly hurt! Anyway, we went back to the room and found out that while I was still at 1 cm (gasp! I know), I was starting to get a little effaced, so that was good! We watched some basketball and then at 11:30 p.m., they came in and started me on Pitocin. The contractions weren't unbearable, and I had always planned on getting an epidural, but after about an hour and a half they started getting really intense. I tried asking for some pain medicine, but the nurse told me that until I dilated more I couldn't have any. She said we should make a goal that I was dilated enough to get the epidural by 7 a.m. This was around 1 a.m., so I was NOT having it. I told her that my goal was to have a baby by 7 a.m., but she told me that wasn't very realistic.

I endured about two and a half more hours of horrible contractions that were about every minute or two and lasted a long time. I kept thinking, "Another one already?" It felt like every time one contraction would end, another would start. I was having a really hard time getting through each contraction, and while I tried to stay positive and nice, I was also unable to find relief in any position I tried. My husband was very supportive and kept asking how he could help, and I tried really hard to focus during each contraction and tell myself that I could do it.

At 3:30 a.m. I finally got some pain medication (although it wasn't the epidural). I'm not sure what it was, but it made me feel loopy and very out of it. I was able to endure the pain better, but it was also hard to open my eyes and focus. I threw up a few times, and after an hour it wore off. I started to think that I couldn't do it, and that I was never going to have my baby. I'm assuming I was more dilated by that point because at 4:30 a.m. I got the epidural. It was hard to sit still while I was having contractions (which I had no idea about), but once it was in it worked like a charm. I was able to relax and I felt so much better.

My husband and I both took little naps for about an hour, and when I woke up at 6 a.m., the nurses checked to see how dilated I was. I'm not sure how far I was, but they told me that they were going to start getting everything ready for our little guy! I distinctly remember after they set up the newborn station and I saw that tiny little baby diaper that would be our baby's very first diaper, I just started bawling. Nine months is a long time to wait to meet your baby, and it was finally almost time!

I don't know exactly what time my water broke, but I had two new nurses at that point so I'm assuming it was some time after 7 a.m. They wanted me to try to break my water on my own, so they helped me get my legs into the stirrups, and when a contraction hit, I pushed. My water popped (like literally popped) all over the older nurse's arms. I felt bad but didn't know if that was normal, so I was like, "I'm sure that's not the first time that's happened." She looked at me and said, "Oh, it's happened one or two times before." Yikes. Apparently, that does not happen very often! Anyway, there was meconium in the fluid so they had the NICU team come down to check him out when he was born.

At this point we were ready to go. My epidural was perfect because I was able to feel pressure and I knew it was time to push, but I couldn't feel any pain. I could wiggle my toes and sort of lift my right leg, and it was just enough feeling that I could have a great delivery. I think it was probably around 7:45 a.m. or so when everyone was there and it was time to push. My doctor told me to push through a contraction and I did, and there was his head! She was trying to tell me to slow down, but there was no way I was going to stop pushing that baby out. After two more contractions and pushes, Jameson Daniel Johnson was born at 7:53 a.m!

Jameson was crying a ton and had a short umbilical cord, so my husband cut it, and then the nurses took him to be checked out on the other side of the room while my doctor sewed me up. His birth happened so fast and I tore pretty long, but not very deep.

My husband was the first person Jameson saw when he opened his eyes (which he still brags about). After they cleaned him up and weighed him, they brought him over to me so I could meet him. He was perfect, and it was so worth the long wait of trying to get pregnant and then nine months of pregnancy to have him there in my arms. He weighed 7 lb, 11 oz, and was 19 ½ inches long, and was a wonderful, easy baby. Now he's a wonderful, easy five year old!

September 4, 2014 – The Birth Story of Ava Jane Johnson

Around 31 weeks I started having Braxton Hicks contractions. I didn't have any that soon with Jameson, so it was different and a little scary because we had a lot of traveling to do in July and the beginning of August. We visited all of our extended family in Idaho, Utah, and Colorado, and then my sister got married right at 35 weeks so I could come (since you aren't supposed to fly after that). Once all the traveling was over at 35 weeks, I was ready for our little girl to be born.

We found out at 37 weeks that I was strep B positive, and because I delivered Jameson so fast, the doctors said that I could be induced at 39 weeks just to make sure that I was able to get antibiotics in time and we wouldn't have to worry about baby girl getting sick. I was having so many Braxton Hicks and it was really frustrating when they would be five minutes apart and then just stop, so I said, "Yes, please!"

We scheduled my induction date at my 38 week appointment for September 3rd, and then we pushed it back to the 4th so that my husband could come and be at the hospital the whole time (darn medical school rotations). On Tuesday Jameson and I went to the zoo, and on Wednesday we tried to do every last thing we could together before we added a new little to our family. My mom drove in on Wednesday so she could stay with Jameson while we were at the hospital. On Thursday morning, six days before my due date, we got a call at 6:15 a.m. that the hospital had a room for us and to be there at 7:30 a.m. We got dressed, had some breakfast, and headed to the hospital.

After we were all checked in and everything was ready to go at 8:30 a.m., I was started on a dose of Pitocin. I was at 1 cm before starting the induction, so I had a lot of work to do! They kept increasing my dosage because while I was having contractions, they weren't doing anything to my cervix. Around 12:30 p.m., they stopped increasing the dosage because they started getting painful. They still weren't bad, but the dosage must've been a good amount because they kept getting worse.

At 2:05 p.m. my doctor came in and broke my water. My contractions were getting more and more painful, but not nearly as painful as when I was in labor with Jameson so I could handle it. The nurse kept telling me that I could get my epidural, but it wasn't until 3:35 p.m. that I asked for it. I was never in too much pain, and the epidural worked perfectly. Unfortunately, I wasn't dilating very quickly, so they turned up my dosage of Pitocin again. After a while, they turned it down again because my contractions were getting too close together and I wasn't dilated enough.

My mom brought Jameson to the hospital around 7 p.m. We couldn't go a whole day without seeing our little boy! Right before they got there I was 5 cm dilated. They were there for a while, and then the nurse turned up my dosage again. After about 20–30 minutes I felt a very strong pressure. The nurse came in and told me I was at 10cm and I was ready to push! My mom and Jameson went out into the lobby, the doctor came in, I pushed through a few contractions, and Ava was born at 8:10 p.m!

Ava had a ton of dark hair, which really surprised us because Jameson was super blonde. She weighed 7 lb, 10 oz, and was 21 inches long, so a little longer than Jameson, but she weighed an ounce less. I got to hold her right after she was born, before she was all cleaned and weighed and everything.

While I was holding her and in new mama bliss, my doctor was trying to get my placenta out. A little bit had been retained, and she had to scrape my uterus to get it all out, which even with an epidural was still kind of painful. I was also bleeding a ton, a fact which I didn't even know until the next day when they told me they had thought I was going to need a transfusion because of all the blood I had lost. My immediate postpartum wasn't quite as simple as it was with my first baby, but I eventually stopped bleeding and was sewn up and everything was fine.

My mom brought Jameson in around 8:40 p.m. and he got to meet his new baby sister. The first thing he did, without us even telling him to, was lean over and kiss her and then pat her. It just melted my mama heart. Your first child always seems so little until your second is born, and then you see them together and realize how big your oldest really is. It warms your heart and breaks it all at the same time.

It took us a whole day to name Ava. Our top choice of names was Ava, but we had been expecting a blonde baby, so when she was born with all that dark hair, we weren't sure if that was still her name. We thought about Lily for a while (Jameson and Lily, like James and Lily Potter!), but after sleeping on it, we settled on Ava. We were able to go home from the hospital two days later, and she's now a happy, super silly three year old!

January 29, 2017 – The Birth Story of Russell Steven Johnson

From day one, I knew I didn't want to be induced with this baby. I had never felt what it was like to actually go into labor on my own, and I knew that I wanted to try my best to not get induced this time. I had been having Braxton Hicks since about halfway through pregnancy, so I thought maybe that was a good sign. I also had planned on trying not to complain as much as I had with my first two pregnancies, but my third pregnancy was rough. By the end, I could barely walk around the house, sit on the floor, or even roll over in bed. To say I was miserable would be an understatement.

So about 10 days before my due date, my husband and I agreed to start trying to get things going. We were hoping that this time it would be different. On Wednesday, he got off of work early so we went and walked/hiked at a local park and had lunch at a spicy Mongolian grill. I also had my membranes stripped and bounced on my friend's exercise ball for a few hours in the evening. That night, I woke up in the middle of the night with contractions that felt more real and were about 10 minutes apart. They weren't super painful yet, but I felt that they were a little more than Braxton Hicks. I got my hopes up, but after a few hours they went away (prodromal labor is the pits). It was a bummer.

On Thursday I did a bunch of bouncing on the exercise ball again, and pretty much thought about going into labor the whole day. It was really stressful, but that night I lost my mucus plug and started getting excited again. Alas, nothing happened.

On Friday the Braxton Hicks came and went throughout the day, and I bounced on the ball several times, too. That night I had prodromal labor again like I did on Wednesday night. Again, it went away.

On Saturday I was feeling pretty frustrated because I felt like something should be happening but nothing was. I tried to relax and didn't do any bouncing or walking or spicy food eating. My husband gave me a massage in the afternoon to help me relax, and even though I usually hate massages, it helped!

On Sunday morning (January 29th, 39 weeks exactly) I woke up at 4:00 a.m. with contractions again. I thought they might be prodromal labor, so I tried not to get my hopes up. I started timing them and they were about 10 minutes apart. Around 7:30 a.m. I got up to go to the bathroom and had a little bloody show. I shouted to my husband what had happened, and even though I was trying to stay calm, I felt my excitement rising again. I kept timing the contractions because I could feel them in my belly and in my back, and they just kept coming, even though I was walking around and drinking water and doing everything you're supposed to do when you think you might be in labor.

We decided to go to church (aka, I decided because I didn't want to sit at home and think about going into labor or not going into labor). We had made the mistake of telling our kids that baby might be coming today, so Jameson kept telling people at church that our baby was going to be born that day. I'm pretty sure they didn't believe him because a) I was there, and b) the day was half over. The contractions kept coming the whole time we were there, and by the end of the three hours, they were about 7–8 minutes apart and I was having to brace myself and breathe through them (imagine that in your Sunday School class!).

When we got home we decided that it was probably time to go to the hospital because I was bending over and stopping what I was doing when the contractions hit. I gathered up the rest of the stuff for my hospital bag, and my husband fed the kids some lunch before we dropped them off at our friends' house and headed to the hospital.

We got there about 1:30 p.m. and when we checked into the triage, it took them a while to get the doctor so he could check me. The contractions were still coming, but they were about eight minutes apart, so I started feeling pretty discouraged. When I was checked at 2:00 p.m., I was 4 cm dilated, which was promising because I'd only ever been 1 cm the whole time before I was induced with Jameson and Ava. They did an ultrasound just to make sure everything looked good and baby boy was head down and measuring about 8½ pounds. We asked if we could walk around the L&D floor to try to get things to progress more (I had to be at 5 cm to get admitted, and a big part of me kept thinking that we were still going to get sent home), so we walked in circles around the floor while I ate ice chips and we tried not to focus on going home.

The contractions kept getting stronger and more painful, and by 4:30 p.m. I was having to stop and double over while holding onto my husband for each one. They hurt a lot, so we decided to go get checked again. I was 5 cm and 50% effaced, so we were told that we were going to get a room, and we were going to have our baby! They also said that if we wanted to wait a little bit, they were cleaning the big room they had (which, honestly, wasn't that big in retrospect), so we decided to wait. We got into the room at 5:15 p.m. and the anesthesiologist was there and ready. I got my epidural at 5:25 p.m., not a moment too soon because at that point I was having a really hard time getting through each contraction.

After I got my epidural, it really hit me that we were going to meet our little boy soon, and I started crying because I was so excited (and so ready to not be pregnant anymore). My husband and I just hung out in the room for a while and then at 7:40 p.m. I was checked again. I was at 7 cm and was 100% effaced. As soon as the nurse finished checking me my water broke and there was a little bit of meconium in it, so they arranged to have the NICU people in the room just to make sure baby was okay right after he was born.

After about 20 minutes, I felt pressure and knew that it was about time to push, so we told the nurse and they called the doctor and got everything ready for baby to be born. My epidural was starting to wear off a little, so I felt everything stretching while he was coming out (it wasn't awful, but it for sure hurt). Because our first two kids were born very quickly, and I only pushed for a few minutes with each of them, I was hoping to do the same with this baby. When we told the nurses that, I don't think they really believed me. Luckily, it only took pushing through three contractions before Russell was born at 8:33 p.m.

My husband cut the umbilical cord while I tried to breathe and catch my breath. The NICU people were in the room, so they checked him out and weighed him and everything before handing him to me. He was 8 lb, 7 oz (my biggest baby by almost a pound), 20¼ inches long, and he was born with a full head of long, dark hair and his daddy's chin.

We were trying to decide between Russell and Hudson for his name, and after a few hours we settled on Russell. We had actually thought about naming Jameson Russell because we watched an Oklahoma City Thunder game while I was in labor with him, and Russell Westbrook was on FIRE that night! But we saved it, and it's the perfect name for our second little guy. His middle name is Steven, which was my father-in-law's name. He passed away when Jameson was 10 months old, and we've always wanted to give one of our children his name.

We had to stay at the hospital until Tuesday because I hadn't had the antibiotics for strep B long enough before he was born (annoying), and the kids came to visit twice on Monday. They kept saying how baby brother was "so cute" and Jameson just wanted to hold him the whole time. It was really special to have just the five of us there together, and it was a great way to begin the transition to having three kids.

I don't know if it's because I got him out quickly and only had a first degree tear, because by the end of pregnancy I could barely move, or because this was my third time going through childbirth, but I recovered really quickly

192

this time around. Physically I felt great, and I didn't even have to sit on that donut thing after, which was awesome because I had three crazy kids to take care of!

1. Callahan, Tamara L., and Aaron B. Caughey. *Obstetrics and gynecology*. 6th ed., Lippincott Williams & Wilkins, 2013.
2. "Placenta previa." *March of Dimes*, Jan. 2012, www.marchofdimes.org/complications/placenta-previa.aspx.
3. Callahan, Tamara L., and Aaron B. Caughey. *Obstetrics and gynecology*. 6th ed., Lippincott Williams & Wilkins, 2013.

Advice

I know that having three kids doesn't make me a parenting expert. I'm constantly learning new things every day (like how potty training is not the same with every child!), and some days I feel like I am completely messing up my kids. And I also know that when you're pregnant or have a new baby, you get a lot of advice. Lots of moms, grandmas, friends, and even strangers will tell you to do things, not do things, what worked for them, and what didn't work for them.

The last section in this book has a few tips for mamas that I hope you'll really think about and take to heart. That being said, I'm not going to be offended if you decide that one of these doesn't really apply to you. We are all different, and we all mother different ways (which is great because how boring would it be if all our kids turned out the same!).

Here's a little new mama advice from me to you:

1. Find what works for you. Like I said, new moms always get tons of advice. Some of it is good, and some of it is bad. One thing a lot of people told me was to nap when

my baby was napping. I'm sure for some people that's good advice, but I've never been much of a napper, so napping while my baby was napping just wasn't good advice for me. So, find out which advice works for you, and forget about the rest. Every baby is different, and every mom is different. Embrace it, and don't worry if a piece of advice isn't for you.

2. You are amazing even if the house is a mess and dinner isn't ready. Sometimes you don't get everything done that you want to. Some days feel like they last forever, and when your husband finally comes home, your house might look like an atomic bomb went off with laundry everywhere. On those days, you might have to order a pizza. And that really is no big deal. You are a mom. You are doing a super hard job, and you are rocking it. So, if you have a day where you don't get everything done on your to-do list, it's okay. You're doing the best you can, and you are amazing.

3. Ask for help if you need it. If you feel overwhelmed by staying home all day with your tiny little baby, ask for help! Ask for a friend or family member to come visit and help out. If you need someone to come over for a bit so you can pee or sit at the table and eat without holding your baby, then ask! It's totally okay to need some help. Being a mom is not something that you get the hang of overnight (and even once you feel like you're doing a good job, something new will happen and you'll be like, "How do I even handle this!?").

4. Write things down. Dates, questions for the doctor, things you don't want to forget, and funny things your kids do. I keep a memory journal for each of my kids, and I write down special memories, milestones, and things I want to remember about them: first smile, first laugh, the

day they started crawling, funny things they say or do. Write things down! Something I have learned as a mom is that your memory gets worse with each child (I am the worst at this), and if I don't write something down, it's likely to be forgotten. So, write things down because later you will want to remember.

5. It's okay to watch them while they sleep. Your baby is going to be the most adorable, beautiful, perfect little person in the whole world. So naturally, you are going to want to watch your baby all the time. I still like to sneak into my kids' rooms and watch them sleep. And that's totally okay! There are few things cuter than a sleeping baby (especially on those rough days where they drive you crazy!).

6. Always say, "I love you." I try to always tell my kids "I love you" before naps or bedtime, even to little baby Russell, who has no idea what that means because he's a baby. I want my kids to always know how I feel about them, and starting early is one way to get it into their little heads!

7. Enjoy naptime. And don't feel guilty if you love naptime. Babies are incredible and you love them with all of your heart, but I think God gave us naps so that we could take little breaks throughout the day. Naptime is one of the only times in the day that you can do things without holding a baby or without being interrupted, so enjoy it while it lasts.

8. Listen to your heart. I know that sort of sounds cheesy, but seriously if you think something is wrong, go check on your baby. If you don't feel good about doing something someone has suggested, don't do it. You know your baby better than anyone else, so you are the one who gets to

make the final decision on things. If something doesn't feel right, don't ignore that feeling. Listen to it.

9. Find a hobby outside of mothering. Motherhood is incredible and the best job I've ever had, but if you don't have a hobby then you are going to get burned out pretty fast. Blogging is my thing that I love to do, and it helps challenge me and keep me on my toes. Of course, motherhood does that too, but I can't tell you how helpful it is to have a hobby or job or something else that you love to do. It's good for your sanity to have something that is "your thing" and I strongly suggest figuring out what that is. It might take a while to figure it out, but keep trying new things! You'll find it!

10. You aren't a bad mom. I saw a quote once that said, "You aren't a bad mom. You are a good mom having a bad day." Sometimes we are going to have bad days where we just sit around and let our kids watch TV and eat snacks. That's okay! Not every day is going to be filled with playgrounds and educational activities and building things out of blocks. Bad days happen, especially to moms, and it's important not to get hung up when they do. Just get through the day, and start the next one off better. You want what is best for your children and that makes you a good mom, even if you have a hard day. And in my experience, children are incredibly forgiving and don't hold grudges, so you can always try harder and do better the next day.

11. Pay attention to yourself. Be aware that postpartum depression happens to a lot of people. If you don't enjoy doing things, if you aren't as happy as you thought you would be with your new baby, if you don't feel like talking to people, or you feel down for longer than two weeks, step outside your situation and realize what is

197

happening. Get help before it gets worse. It's nothing to be ashamed of, and more people suffer from postpartum depression than you know. So, pay attention to yourself, and if you think you might be struggling with PPD, get help.

12. Don't take pictures of everything. Yes, your baby is the cutest thing in the world and no baby has ever been cuter. But you don't need to capture every single moment on camera. It's way more important to be there in the moment than to take a picture of every moment. When I realized that I didn't need to take a million pictures of my kids, it was actually pretty freeing. I want to enjoy the moments I have with my kids face-to-face instead of being behind the lens of my camera or the screen of my smartphone.

13. Disconnect. I think social media is ruining family time. I don't want my children to grow up thinking that Mommy and Daddy are always on their phones. So, when you are with your baby, be with your baby, not half with them and half on Facebook. Social media is great for some things, and I think it's a great way to share photos of your baby with family who live far away and to connect with other mamas, but don't get caught up in wasting time scrolling through photos and statuses of people you haven't seen since high school (or people you've never even met!). Who cares what they're doing? Your kids need you, and putting your phone in a different room while you are with them isn't going to be something you regret.

14. Love your body. You just pushed a baby out of your body. Go you! Your tummy is going to be baggy and squishy, you are going to feel flabby all over, and it's going to take time before those varicose veins go away.

Jell-O tummies happen to every new mom. Your body is incredible. There was a human baby inside of you for nine months! Of course your body is going to look and feel a little funny at first. But be patient, and be grateful for what your amazing body has done. Be nice to it and don't get down on yourself.

15. Remember that everyone is different. Everyone's pregnancy is different, everyone's birth is different, and everyone's postpartum is different. Babies are different, they grow at different rates, and they achieve milestones at different ages. Theodore Roosevelt once said, "Comparison is the thief of joy," and it absolutely applies to motherhood. Don't compare yourself, your pregnancy, or your baby to someone else's. That's not fair to you or your child.

If one of these tips doesn't work for you, I promise I'm not offended. You are different than me, and that's awesome. So, congratulations on your pregnancy, becoming a new mama, and for finishing this book! Being a mom is the best thing in the world, and you're going to love it!

Thanks

I have so many people that I could thank, but I want to first of all thank my Heavenly Father for giving me my writing talent, for the blessing of getting pregnant and giving birth to three healthy babies, for helping me finish this book despite getting pregnant again and having three kids to take care of, and for innumerable other blessings that I could fill a whole second book with if I wrote them all down.

Thank you to my husband, Dan, who keeps impregnating me, for his unwavering support, for his hard work in supporting our family, and for keeping our kids busy and out of the office so I could finish writing my book. He's my perfect match in every way imaginable, and I love him with all of my heart.

Thank you to my mom for getting pregnant with me, for giving birth to me, and for raising me. Thank you for your encouragement, for supporting me in whatever new thing I've wanted to try, and for letting me figure things out on my own so I could grow into who I am today.

Thank you to my dad for giving me an X chromosome so I could get pregnant one day, for his friendship and love, and for talking to me on the phone whenever I want someone to talk to.

Thank you to my little sister, Becca, and to my best friend, Melissa, who didn't laugh when I told them I was writing a book, who read parts of my book before I shared it with anyone else, and who are always supportive of whatever I do. And thanks to my other friends Marci and Bekah who also read my book before it was finished and gave me great feedback.

Thank you to my mother-in-law, Kim, and my father-in-law, Steve, for getting married and making the most amazing man I have ever met.

Thank you to my college roommate, Kirsten, who used her editing minor and edited my book before I published it.

Thank you to Steph Hansen for taking pictures in my backyard of my pregnant belly in front of a bright pink wooden board that I painted so that my book cover would be exactly how I imagined it from day one.

Thank you to all the readers of my blog who showed me that people would actually read what I wrote and who continue to visit my blog, even after four years of posts.

And last of all, thanks to you for reading my book. I'll be honest and tell you I cried a little bit when I finished writing it because it took almost two years, it was really hard, and it's actually a huge deal to me. The fact that you picked it up, decided to read it, and actually read the whole thing means the world to me. So thank you.

About the Author

Chelsea Johnson was born and raised in Colorado. After moving to Utah for college, she met her husband Dan, and eleven months later they were married. She graduated from Brigham Young University with a bachelor's degree in Family Life with an emphasis in Family Studies and a minor in Anthropology. In 2013 she started writing *Life With My Littles*, her blog all about pregnancy and parenting. It steadily grew and has become a popular mommy blog for new and seasoned moms alike. Chelsea loves Harry Potter, pizza, running, and the color pink. She and her husband Dan currently live in Minnesota with their three children.

Connect With Me

My Blog: *Life With My Littles*, www.lifewithmylittles.com

Facebook: www.facebook.com/lifewmylittles

Pinterest: www.pinterest.com/littleschelsea

Instagram: www.instagram.com/lifewmylittles

Twitter: www.twitter.com/lifewmylittles

Preggers Website: www.preggersthebook.com

Preggers Instagram: www.instagram.com/preggersthebook